Thyroid Mind Power

Thyroid Mind Power

The Proven Cure for Hormone-Related Depression, Anxiety, and Memory Loss

Richard Shames, MD,
and Karilee Shames, PhD, RN
with Georjana Grace Shames, LAc

RODALE

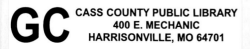

Rodale books may be purchased for business or promotional use or for special sales. For information, please write to:
Special Markets Department, Rodale Inc., 733 Third Avenue, New York, NY 10017

Printed in the United States of America
Rodale Inc. makes every effort to use acid-free ∞, recycled paper ♻.

Illustrations by Brian Narelle
briannarelle.com

Book design by Kara Plikaitis

Library of Congress Cataloging-in-Publication Data

Shames, Richard.
    Thyroid mind power : the proven cure for hormone-related depression, anxiety, and memory loss / Richard Shames and Karilee Shames, with Georjana Grace Shames.
        p.   cm.
    Includes bibliographical references.
    ISBN 978-1-60529-278-6   paperback
    1. Hypothyroidism—Popular works.   I. Shames, Karilee Halo.   II. Shames, Georjana Grace.   III. Title.
RC657.S52   2010
616.4'44—dc22   2010040642

Distributed to the trade by Macmillan
2   4   6   8   10   9   7   5   3   1   paperback

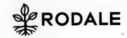

We inspire and enable people to improve their lives and the world around them.
www.rodalebooks.com

Contents

Foreword by Sam Von Reiche, PsyD   vii

Acknowledgments   x

Introduction   xi

An Invitation from the Authors   xxi

PART I: Consider a Thyroid Cause

Chapter 1:   Missing the Boat on Mind-Body Connections   3

Chapter 2:   Thyroid Imbalance Often Causes Mental Imbalance   27

Chapter 3:   Is Thyroid Causing YOUR Symptoms?   51

PART II: Understand Your Best Treatment

Chapter 4:   The MOODY Mind-Type: Overcome Depression, Mood Swings, and Negative Thinking   75

Chapter 5:   The EDGY Mind-Type: Reduce Anxiety, Panic, Irritability, Anger, and Rage   105

Chapter 6:   The FOGGY Mind-Type: Improve Attention Deficit, Memory Loss, and Dementia   137

Chapter 7:   The SLEEPY Mind-Type: Relieve Insomnia, Narcolepsy, and Nonrefreshing Sleep   159

Chapter 8:   The NEEDY Mind-Type: Recover from Eating Disorders, Substance Abuse, and Addiction   185

PART III: **Maintain a Lasting Cure**

Chapter 9:   Enhance Your Thyroid Treatment: Add Vitamins,
             Minerals, Herbs, Acupuncture, and Oriental Medicine   209

Chapter 10: Enjoy a More Powerful Lifestyle: Making Time for
             Nutrition, Stress Reduction, Exercise, Bodywork,
             and Spirituality   225

The Program in a Nutshell   261

Afterword   265

Appendix   273

  Self-Ordering Your Own Accurate Thyroid Tests   273

  Finding and Working with
  Thyroid-Friendly Practitioners   275

  Finding Your Recommended Vitamins   279

Resources   281

Notes and References   285

Index   292

Foreword

*Woven within the tapestry of professional development
are always our threads of personal challenge, and discovery.*

The story of how I came to collaborate with Drs. Rich and Karilee Shames began with my own bout of mysterious illness in 2001.

Looking back, I was probably moderately hypothyroid since childhood, experiencing symptoms such as inordinate depression and fatigue, while most other kids were bouncing happily around the neighborhood.

My hands and feet were always, and I mean *always*, unexplainably cold. Because my father had similar symptoms, I figured it was just genetic and did my best to cope through the early part of my life.

When my forties came around, however, it was a different story. Suddenly, I gained more than 20 pounds on my slender frame without explanation. I was so exhausted I could barely get through the day and would lapse into comalike naps every chance I got.

I felt so depressed and anxious I cried and worried obsessively every day.

So much of my hair fell out I actually had nightmares about it, while my hands and feet constantly felt like I had been thrown into a meat locker for a day.

Totally desperate, I consulted with many of my medical colleagues. I was tested for everything from anemia to leukemia, but to no avail.

Having heard somewhere that weight gain could be caused by low thyroid, I asked for thyroid testing. The singular standard TSH test came back "within normal limits." Perhaps like many of you reading this, I was assured that there was "absolutely nothing wrong" with my thyroid.

Chalking my plethora of perplexing symptoms up to stress, and my slowing metabolism to age, my well-meaning colleagues dismissed me—shockingly and completely. I was still so sick.

Sensing on a gut level that my thyroid was making me ill, I resorted to reading every book on the subject at Barnes and Noble. I thank my lucky stars that the Shames's book *Thyroid Power* was one of them, because there began my healing journey.

Based on their evaluation and suggestions, I concluded that I was indeed hypothyroid and requested additional tests. I was shocked back then at the resistance of my conventional medical colleagues (including acquaintances and friends) to simply order further testing.

They insisted the TSH test was "exquisitely sensitive" and that I (of course) was being stubborn.

If it hadn't been for the Shames's book, I might have given up. Finally, I was able to convince one colleague to give me the two thyroid antibody tests, which came back grossly abnormal.

Amazingly, even then my lovely primary care physician insisted the tests did not mean I was hypothyroid! After much arguing and begging, she prescribed the lowest dose of Synthroid, and the rest, shall we say, is history.

On the second day of taking medication, it was as though the heavens opened up for me. I opened my eyes without a struggle for the first time in months. A diagnosis of Hashimoto's thyroiditis eventually followed.

With the change to a T3/T4 medication (also endorsed by Dr. Shames) and a significant dosage increase, I was back to myself again within a few months. My depression and obsessive worrying had disappeared; my energy level had rebounded, in generous supply.

Happily, I returned to my normal weight, managing to fit back into my clothes with a deep sense of relief. There was so much that improved, it seemed impossible that one little pill could make such a huge difference. I had at last regained the Self I hadn't been since I was 11 years old.

My thyroid cure was radically life changing on many levels. I became an enthusiastic advocate of mind-body healing, both in my own life and in my practice.

I began to focus on this overlooked role of thyroid issues in psychological health. Over the next 10 years, I eventually identified more than 200 cases of hidden hypothyroidism that had been causing persistent mental symptoms in my patients, colleagues, friends, and family members.

The greatest stories of all belong to our patients. All too often they had wandered from one therapist to another in the seemingly endless struggle to figure out what was wrong with them. Now, many are finally doing much better with good thyroid care.

Regards and best wishes for your success as well,
Sam Von Reiche, PsyD,
Clinical Psychologist and Success Coach
Clifton, New Jersey

Acknowledgments

We are exceedingly grateful to the large number of people involved in bringing our thyroid work to publication. We especially want to thank:

- Our devoted colleagues and hardworking staff at the Preventive Medicine Center of Marin in San Rafael, California
- Those many openhearted and insightful patients who have offered us their feedback and inspiration
- The researchers and epidemiologists who are diligently uncovering the many interconnections in this complex field
- Faith Hamlin, our amazing agent at Sanford Greenberger Associates, for her continued focus on key health issues
- Shannon Welch, our delightful editor at Rodale Inc., for her remarkable clarity and support and Stephanie Knapp, Editorial Assistant
- Georgia Kahn, this book's manuscript consultant, for her careful adherence to detail and deadlines
- Lynn Larkin, dedicated Canary Club founder (www.CanaryClub.org), for helping many thyroid sufferers to finally get their true diagnosis
- Mary Shomon, thyroid advocate par excellence, for her open-hearted support of our efforts
- Brian Narelle, master cartoonist, who brings ideas into form (NarelleCreative.net; briannarelle@comcast.net)

Introduction

You may be shocked to discover how thyroid balance affects your mind.

When some of the 40 million Americans with thyroid imbalance manage to see *endocrine doctors*, these specialists are not at all surprised to find symptoms of depression, anxiety, memory loss, sleep problems, or even excessive cravings. Such symptoms are commonly a direct mental result of the thyroid's effect on brain chemistry.

These psychological symptoms often resolve with good thyroid care.

But when the majority of these same 40 million, with their same mental symptoms, see *primary care practitioners*, something different happens.

They are often given a mental diagnosis, prescribed an antidepressant medicine, and referred to a psychiatrist.

This is even more likely if the causative thyroid problem is not the kind that shows up easily on one simple, overrated blood test. Researchers estimate that half of all thyroid problems are undiagnosed.

Misdiagnosing thyroid imbalance as a mental problem is quite costly.

- Expensive psychological medicines and lengthy psychotherapy can never fully resolve the underlying physical issue of gland dysfunction.
- Missing the true diagnosis can lead to years of untreated hyper- or hypothyroidism.
- This in turn leads to increased amounts of diabetes, heart disease, weight gain, and infertility.

All of this—and more—would greatly improve if practitioners and patients alike could just be more aware of the commonly occurring **thyroid connection to mental health.**

This Began as a Personal Quest

It started when Karilee was diagnosed at age 20 with Hashimoto's thyroiditis, a very common inflammation of the thyroid gland affecting tens of millions of Americans. She had struggled with this condition for several decades, often not receiving the kind of care she knew was possible.

It turned out that what many doctors consider boring and routine was something we became passionate about, the accurate diagnosis and creative treatment of mild thyroid imbalance. It quickly became crystal clear to us as medical professionals that millions are suffering needlessly and also that we, an integrative doctor-nurse team, could help them to improve their lives.

What began for us as a personal quest has evolved into our mission: to help you reclaim your greatest health and enjoyment of your life.

How Is This Book Different?

Some of you may have read our earlier books, *Thyroid Power* and *Feeling Fat, Fuzzy, or Frazzled?* Each was our attempt to further demystify complex hormonal issues related to thyroid balance in a way that would empower health consumers to take back their lives and reclaim their health.

Thyroid Power introduced the importance of thyroid balancing with a 10-step program to reclaim better thyroid health. Then *Feeling Fat, Fuzzy, or Frazzled?* added a three-gland balancing program to restore thyroid, adrenal, and sex gland balance. Now we invite you to take another step forward on the journey. Here we are moving to another realm, beyond the physical to the mental.

This exploration may help those who are feeling fat or frazzled, but the **focus now is on how to improve your attitude and relationships**. This book offers some very personal perspectives that we hope will help you to better understand your own emotional conditions, whether you have diagnosed mental health issues or not.

Who Will This Book Help?

- For those who have read books about thyroid, this book is unique in its focus on restoring mental well-being.

- For those who have sought self-improvement from "mind power" books, this book can augment and enhance your endeavors to improve your mental health.

- For those with a family history of mental disorders, this book can help you to restore greater balance to yourself and your lineage.

- For those who feel they could benefit from greater mental health, no matter to what degree it may be affecting your life, this book can help.

This book is for anyone who seeks greater mental health.

It is specifically written for those who may be functioning reasonably but seek new ways to improve their mood and behaviors, so they can enjoy more peace and productivity in their lives. It also is written for those with diagnosed mental problems in themselves or loved ones, to minimize uncomfortable symptoms, helping to improve their quality of daily life.

The "Walking Well"

If you **seek greater balance and success**, you may want to consider whether you can restore your biochemical balance to improve your life.

If you are functioning, but **want to feel better and perform better**, you may wish to explore whether your thyroid is out of balance. Sluggish thyroid function can cause mental fatigue and memory and mood problems that can often be easily remedied.

If you struggle with **undiagnosed or undertreated thyroid problems**, you may indeed be able to feel much better. Your attempts at restoring mental health can be enhanced by addressing the biochemical aspects of mood *along with* ingrained patterns of behavior and attitude.

Some of our patterns of behavior arose in our early lives, becoming solidified as we resorted to them again and again. It can be tricky to determine whether your actions are a result of compulsive repetition (treating others as you were treated when young, such as occurs with familial abuse) or whether they are a result of a recent hormonal imbalance.

The good news is: either way, these mental results of physical imbalance can be consciously improved, in the simple steps presented here.

Let's face it: most of us have developed patterns of behavior we would like to change—if we only could. Some of us may have been trying for years to feel and act better via self-improvement and psychotherapy, often without reaching the success we desired.

If you have noticed uncomfortable fluctuations in your mood or mental outlook (including those related to the effects of excessive stress, family dysfunction, or dietary intake), you can learn to become a better master of these emotions. We believe that change can best happen incrementally, rather than dramatically.

As you begin to restore a better balance to your hormones, your brain function and mental outlook will improve. It may have taken years for you to develop the conditions that have been derailing your enjoyment of life, but fortunately you can now reverse this process fairly quickly. You and your loved ones can now be restored to full mental health.

Our commitment is to walk with you through these dark places, to help you begin to understand how you became this way, and to support you with tools and information to take the steps that will enable you to feel your best.

For Those with Family History of Mental Illness

Too little is said about the effects of mental illness on families. Sadly, we as a culture still hide these conditions in dark corners. This book is intended to shine light on these forgotten lives, to help bring them out of the darkness and into the light.

As practitioners with advanced psychiatric training, we hope to uncover some of the mysteries of mental imbalance, sharing natural approaches to support you in helping your loved ones. If you feel you could be more successful with an improved mental outlook, this book can change your life.

If someone you love has been diagnosed with mental illness (schizophrenia, bipolar disorder, affective disorders, severe neurosis, or major depression), this book may help to alleviate some of the symptoms so they can live better. It may help you to restore yourself as caregiver so you can be more effective, finding more joy in your own life while helping those you love.

It may also create small miracles as you work with those you love, whose welfare may be entrusted to your care. We believe every person on Earth was put here for a purpose, and that helping to rebalance the thyroid can be an important step on the journey to wellness and life's enjoyment. If we can touch one life and help that person to feel better, we will have met our goals.

But Is This Book for *Me*?

You may be saying, "This book is only for those with mental illness."

The truth is that there are many millions more with milder or yet undiagnosed mood problems, who may have some of the symptoms below:

- Inability to be happy
- Depression
- Anxiety
- Cycles of mood elevations and crashes
- Irritability
- Rage
- Addictions
- Sleep disorders
- Autism
- ADD

Who Are We—And Why Did We Write This Book?

Karilee is a master's-prepared certified clinical specialist in Psychiatric Nursing with a PhD in Holistic Studies, in mental health practice for more than 30 years. Richard has worked for more than 30 years as a general medical doctor. Over these decades, we have guided thousands of patients with hormonal imbalance toward restoration of more optimal psychological function.

Over the span of our careers, one of the most surprising benefits of restoring hormone balance has been the associated improvement in previously recalcitrant mental/emotional symptoms. We have seen lives turn around with the simple recommendations offered here.

We wish for you this same healing.

(continued on page xviii)

Karilee's Corner

Florence Nightingale, founder of modern nursing, grew up in Victorian England, where women were exalted for their spirituality while tending the domestic altar. It was a life she loathed. In desperation, she wrote a pamphlet called "Cassandra" in 1852. It is a work of anger and despair.

Cassandra, in Greek mythology, was the daughter of King Priam and Queen Hecuba of Troy. Apollo granted her the gift of prophecy, but later cursed her so that her words would not be believed.

This combination of deep understanding and powerlessness exemplifies the tragic condition of women in most societies.

After her return from the Crimean War, Nightingale became a bedridden invalid. She was described by Sir George Pickering in *Creative Malady*, suggesting her illness was a "psychoneurosis with a purpose."

Indeed, her own words on women's lives give meaning to her inner turmoil: "The accumulation of nervous energy, which has had nothing to do during the day, makes them feel every night, when they go to bed, as if they were going mad . . ."

Historically, women have been susceptible to highly emotional states that seemed to arise from hormonal issues.

- In the time of Hippocrates, and in ancient Greece, there was a condition called *melancholia*, characterized by an unremitting mood of apprehension and gloom. It was much later shown to have increased sleep abnormalities, with less REM sleep, and high night cortisol levels.

- Until the 17th century, *hysteria* was a common diagnosis for women, arising from Hippocrates' suggestion that women's escalated agitation was caused by a womb problem (*hystera* in Greek).

- In the latter 1800s, Jean-Martin Charcot, a French neurologist, advanced the study of this condition, determining after studying nervous conditions that these were hereditary.

- There was also another popular term, *lacissitude,* now called *lassitude,* referring to a deepened ongoing state of exhaustion.

- Once a common psychiatric diagnosis, *neurosis* is a term rarely used today, except in psychoanalytic theory. When originally coined, it was thought to be a nervous system disorder. It refers to functional mental disorders involving distress, without hallucinations or delusions. Carl Jung found that while these individuals could function, they had issues with the meaning of their lives.

While it is clear that women's biochemistry is more complicated than that of males, it is also clear to us, as practitioners since the early 1970s, that *women have not been studied adequately,* nor evaluated carefully enough, to fully understand the many interactions that can be causing problems.

A Jungian analyst related hysteria to the Cassandra Complex, wherein women have emotional or physical suffering, often gynecological, characterized by the women being disbelieved or dismissed.

We have made a decision to write this book in support of all women, and men, facing mental symptoms that can arise from physical situations, specifically disturbance of hormone balance.

We believe the throngs of women—and men—who come through our clinic, complaining of maladies that many doctors quickly assume are "mental." As practitioners each with a 40-year history of mind-body approaches to health, we do not make the distinction between mind and body. Instead, we work with you as a full human being, a combination of body-mind-spirit.

You are a unique person; you deserve unique medicine.

Thyroid imbalance alone can cause a host of mental symptoms, along with its slew of physical symptoms.

It could be that the new terminology for what was previously labeled neurosis, lacissitude, hysteria, or melancholia will be *thyroid imbalance.*

We cannot determine whether a person truly has an organic mental diagnosis until carefully ruling out *a thyroid problem* as the cause for these symptoms.

This book is dedicated to the many women who, like Cassandra, have not been listened to carefully, or heard fully, often by the doctors entrusted with their care.

We are here, listening carefully, eager to support your evolution as your own best healer, physician, and caregiver.

We encourage you to take back your health now, as only you can do.

Complementary Healing for Your Best Results

HELLO, THIS IS ACUPUNCTURIST GEORJANA SHAMES—the daughter of Drs. Richard and Karilee Shames. It is my utmost pleasure to serve as a conduit to the medicine of ancient China for you in this book.

For simplicity's sake, in this book we combine all the practices of Traditional Chinese Medicine into the category of "Acupuncture," but there were many different modalities used in ancient China that can be of great benefit to your thyroid and mental health today.

The practices of acupuncture form an intricate system of modalities rich with 5 millennia of history. These include the insertion of hair-thin needles into specific points on the human body, herbal formulas, medical massage, diet modifications, stress reduction, lifestyle guidance, and more.

Acupuncture has been lauded as the longest-running clinical trial of any medicine, helping approximately *4 billion people* over the past 5,000 years.

How can the practices of acupuncture help you today in your quest for better mental health, especially if you are struggling with a thyroid condition? Many individuals with thyroid imbalances experience symptoms that can be difficult to diagnose and treat successfully. For instance, fatigue, exhaustion, weight gain, hair loss, joint pain, feeling cold constantly, hot flashes, waking multiple times at night, and many other symptoms let us know when our thyroid is not functioning optimally.

But what about the lesser-known symptoms that affect foremost the mental aspects, such as anxiety, depression, lack of mental clarity, obsessive-compulsive disorder, social anxiety disorder, and so on? These can all affect your ability to lead a fulfilling life, and in fact, sometimes they are the only indication of a thyroid condition in the patient.

Actually, I come from a long line of thyroid sufferers. To the best of my knowledge, I could have been considered clinically depressed by the time I was 9 or 10 years old. I was very unhappy in school, overwhelmed by the many activities children often love and look forward to. Birthday parties and social events were stressful for me.

It is quite possible that I was suffering even as a young child from thyroid depletion. Fortunately, by the time I was 13 or 14 years old, I was diagnosed, and put on a high-quality thyroid regimen that includes Chinese Medicine and thyroid medicines, all of which was very helpful to me.

If you feel your current regimen does not quite manage all of your symptoms, you may need to add dietetics, acupuncture, and better thyroid medicine.

We can also learn a whole lot from our suffering, even from the years when our thyroid was out of balance. There are so many benefits of having had this experience; it has helped my practice immensely, as I am able to understand and empathize with thyroid patients I now treat. I have more than just a clinical knowledge of this condition; I also have a personal knowledge of which modalities are the most effective for thyroid care.

Today as an acupuncturist, I work alongside my parents, who have long appreciated the wisdom of both Eastern and Western methods, traditional and alternative practices that are very effective for treating and even curing hormone imbalances. My father long believed the 5,000-year-old system of acupuncture has so much to offer thyroid patients that he strongly encouraged me to pursue this field of medicine professionally. And we are now very pleased to offer the high efficacy of an integrative approach to our patients.

It is the task of every acupuncturist to address the patient on an individual basis, wherein the pillars of Chinese diagnosis, such as pulse and tongue evaluation, lead to treatment protocols that are designed *specifically for you*.

The acupuncturist's goal when he or she stimulates points, or creates herbal formulas for each patient, is to restore balance to the

Chinese Medicine system of energy pathways we call meridians, which crisscross the body in a similar fashion to the lymph or nervous system in Western medicine. In the case of hormone conditions, we work to restore balance to the 14 main meridians and to regulate the affected organ systems that have become weak (whether from genetic predisposition; stress; ingesting pollutants in our air, food, or water; or other causes).

The crux of our medicine is to awaken the body's original intelligence to heal itself.

I look forward to explaining more about the contemporary applications for acupuncture in this book, and how it can help you to cultivate a more balanced and energetic lifestyle.

Included in each chapter of this book is a section I have added, called "Complementary Healing for Your Best Results." I hope this enriches your experience and helps you to improve your health.

An Invitation from the Authors on Special Assistance and Coaching

For those who can use our written suggestions to balance your own hormones by yourself, we say to you, **"Good going!"**

For those who could use more hands-on help, we have created an option just for you!

Many people opt to do at least **one telephone coaching session with your author Dr. Rich Shames** before seeking a local thyroid practitioner.

This can easily be arranged by downloading the "Coaching Agreement Form" from our website, www.ThyroidMindPower.com.

- He will spend an hour on the phone with you, helping you to **understand exactly what may be going on** with your hormones.
- During this session, he will take your health history and **explain your test results**. (After you make your appointment, you can fax over any recent test results or notes that you write up for him.)
- He advises you about **how to speak to your doctor** to get more of what you need.
- **If you do not have a local doctor** to work with on your thyroid issues, **Dr. Shames can make recommendations** from our database for your area, after hearing more about your situation.
- He can also help you to **properly begin your jump start** and integrative therapies program at this time. Many people feel better just starting on the right products for their mind-type.

If anxiety, depression, irritability, or rage is among your issues, you may also wish to engage in some psychotherapy for a while, until your hormones are better balanced.

Or **you can schedule a telephone coaching session with your nurse psychotherapist author, Karilee Shames, PhD, RN**, for easy tips on how to feel better while in the process of thyroid hormone balancing. She can help you learn to meditate, visualize, breathe, and be more aware of your body's messages. Karilee is available for a variety of health coaching needs.

You are also welcome to make a telephone or in-person appointment through our office with Georjana Shames for acupuncture, nutritional consultation, or complementary medicine support. She is particularly adept at isolating the one ingredient that is sometimes missing in an otherwise successful program.

Please review our website for simple directions on how to schedule an in-office appointment or telephone session at www.ThyroidMindPower.com/Appointments.

After that, contact our medical office at 415–388–0456 to schedule your appointment. (Our office is busy, yet dedicated to serving your needs.) Thank you for your patience.

Please note: We are able to help you find local practitioners and give advice about your personal medical situation *only in the context of a telephone coaching session*.

We look forward to getting to know you and supporting your evolution to wholeness. It will be our pleasure to serve your health needs.

PART I

Consider a Thyroid Cause

Thyroid imbalance is one of the most common and misdiagnosed of all physical conditions. The number of prescriptions for thyroid medicines exceeds that for almost any other category of illness. Thus, the chance that you might have a thyroid issue is well worth considering, even if you have "normal" tests.

If you have troublesome mental symptoms and have not been diagnosed with a thyroid problem, we present here a straightforward way to determine whether thyroid imbalance might be an issue for you.

If you have already been diagnosed with a thyroid problem but are still having mental symptoms in spite of thyroid treatment, you may need better thyroid care.

This first section addresses these concerns, helping you to decide when to seek further attention for your thyroid.

1

Missing the Boat on Mind-Body Connections

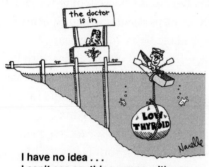

I have no idea . . .
I can't see anything wrong with you.

It is often said: "Low thyroid doesn't kill you, it just makes you wish you were dead."

But, occasionally, it *can* kill.

> Her long-standing anxiety had escalated into uncontrollable panic. The dean's mother was then hospitalized and soon transferred to a mental unit. There, after several agitated episodes, she fell, hit her head, and died.
>
> As dean of the School of Nursing, Dr. Templin requested a case review and autopsy. Only then was it discovered that the reason for her mother's distress was *simple untreated low thyroid*. Had they originally performed better testing, she might have avoided months of terror, enjoying her family for years to come. Dr. Templin's sadness was evident, as was her guilt.

She later lamented: "If I, as professor of nursing for all these years, missed my own mother's true problem, imagine how many other practitioners might be missing the thyroid diagnosis! Think of all the patients suffering with these terrible mental symptoms that could be better controlled with proper thyroid care."

The dean then invited an assistant professor to coauthor an article on better thyroid diagnosis for a major nursing journal.

The assistant professor of nursing was Karilee Shames, PhD, RN. And that article inspired *Thyroid Mind Power*.

Thyroid conditions are surprisingly common, representing possibly the largest category of sufferers in the country. How could the most common of all conditions be so frequently mishandled?

By the late 20th century, thyroid hormones had become the most often prescribed pills. In the early 2000s, one particular brand, Synthroid, was the second most commonly prescribed medicine in America.

Thyroid imbalance is a medical condition that often carries with it a variety of well-studied psychological symptoms. Millions of people face emotional havoc due to simple untreated or poorly treated thyroid imbalances. The health consumers of our country deserve better care.

In this book, we discuss an aspect of health care far too frequently misdiagnosed. It may help to save your life, or at least your *quality* of life, as well as that of people you love.

The Thyroid Gland: Culprit or Cure?

A tiny butterfly-shaped gland at the base of the neck can make our lives heaven or hell. The thyroid, part of our endocrine system, directs our metabolism. It secretes a hormone that drives all of our bodily organs and activities.

Think of your body as a car. The thyroid functions as the gas pedal. It controls the rate and quality of function for every tissue in the body, *including the brain*. A person with severely low thyroid often has the resulting symptoms of low body temperature, slow movements, low heart rate, slow digestion, slow speech, poor sleep, bad memory, slow thoughts, and low mood.

Thus, **thyroid malfunction encompasses aspects of both body and mind**. Keeping the thyroid functioning properly can help millions of people feel better fast. Allowing our thyroids to malfunction is wreaking havoc on our world.

> **Far too many people are living today with low-level or mild thyroid imbalances causing a great deal of chaos in their lives—and wreaking havoc with our lives as well.**

> **To function better as a society, we will need to reorient our focus to enable millions who are feeling tired, depressed, and less than whole to return to a fuller life.**

In our view, fixing the thyroid is one of the easiest and best cures for many problems that ail us. It can be inexpensive and all-encompassing and can greatly improve the quality of life for millions.

The Dangerous Mind-Body Split

In centuries past, scientists and clergy made decisions to separate turf by considering the mind and body as separate entities, operating in totally distinct realms.

In today's world, it remains convenient to continue to adopt this perspective. Many doctors, nurses, health administrators, health insurers, psychologists, counselors, pharmacists, and other providers consider that treating a person's body has very little to do with his mind, and that treating the mind hardly impacts the body. The sad result of this thinking is that we now have specialists and medicines for mental problems, plus separate providers and drugs for physical challenges.

This artificial separation leaves a huge number of hormonally challenged people trapped. Doctors give them medicines for physical symptoms, psychiatrists give them medicines for mental symptoms, and each ignores the hormonal action at the interface of physical and mental. This is unacceptable for the millions experiencing mental challenges due to their physical hormonal condition.

Our culture is looking for quick fixes, but not in the right places. Today's medical system readily employs mind-altering drugs to change our behavior or mood. In many instances, however, this quick fix is not the optimal solution for the longer haul.

In addition to fixing symptoms, we must also make advances in treating the root cause of the condition. Otherwise, many will be doomed to ingest heavy pharmacologic drugs for the rest of their lives.

Surely many of our pharmacologic advances are brilliant and can be helpful when we face crises. Not everyone, however, can afford these costly drugs, and those who can might eventually need other drugs that could interfere with them and cause major problems.

Unless we are attempting *to replace something* the body normally *makes but is deficient in* (due to sluggish production), or *unless we are facing critical illness* without the daily ingestion of a medication, **it is unlikely to be healthy to take pharmacologic medications forever**. Not only do we consider it perhaps unhealthy, but also we often consider it overkill.

Adopting a Perspective of Wholeness

Our goal with our patients has always been to help them gain more confidence in their abilities to heal their own personal pain, to help them minimize the expression of physical pain that can often have psychological underpinnings, and to help them learn to express themselves clearly and effectively.

Our previous books about the thyroid have encouraged people to use their illnesses as an opportunity to learn to heal themselves fully—body, mind, and spirit. We choose to honor the interconnections that make us whole.

Keep in mind that we were young practitioners during the holistic movement of the early 1970s, when the concepts of whole-person treatment were being developed in our country, starting mostly in California, where we live. Richard was a cofounder of one of the first holistic centers in California in the early 1970s. In the mid-1970s, Karilee developed a holistic nursing program there, implementing the concepts of integrative care.

We spend quality time with our patients, inspiring them through our words and personal stories to try our new ways of living. We help them to break free of their fears and to dissociate from the projected fears of their doctors and others less informed. We inspire them to use their own beliefs and intuition in approaching their health challenges. Our central belief honors each person as absolutely the best healer for his or her own health situation. Our way of viewing our patients has been informed by decades of study in sociology, psychology, anthropology and cultural awareness, human behavior, endocrinology, neurology, general medicine, nursing, religion, and various other systems.

Having spent decades thinking as whole-person health professionals, we believe that many of our patients' emotional challenges are best viewed through the hormonal lens. Along with hormone balancing, we have consistently encouraged habit changes coupled with new ways of thinking.

When our first thyroid book came out in 2000, people attending our book signings were upset that we were directing people to get better care from their doctors, because their doctors did not know how to do a good job on thyroid boosting. We realize, sadly, that our way of thinking may not yet be shared by the majority of our colleagues. And herein lies the greater challenge.

A Look at the Science

We don't want to bog you down with a lot of jargon and academic research, but we feel that the best health consumers are educated consumers. With that in mind, we've included a few select research studies in each chapter, with the full reference listed in a chapter-by-chapter list at the end of the book. If you are not interested, feel free to browse forward to the next section.

- The prevalence of thyroid conditions runs from about 5% to almost 25% of the population being studied. While thyroid imbalance is a very common condition among women, men also have thyroid problems, though far less often. (Feit)

- **Thyroid problems also become more common as we age.** The numbers of postmenopausal women who have some degree of thyroid abnormality ranged up to 26% in a 2001 study published in the prestigious *Journal of Epidemiology.*

- In the early 2000s, the Columbia-Presbyterian Medical Center in New York estimated that **more than 20 million people in the United States were currently taking thyroid medicine**. At the time, this figure was believed to be higher than that of all people taking diabetes and cancer medicine *combined*. (Ditkoff)

- Professor Chester Ridgeway at the University of Colorado Health Sciences Center tested more than 25,000 normal people, finding that a surprising percentage of them actually had a hidden thyroid condition. His calculations allowed him to estimate that another **13 million Americans with some degree of hypothyroidism would be detected** by simply having a TSH test. (Ridgeway)

- In 2002 the American Association of Clinical Endocrinologists (AACE) published information suggesting that many more people would be properly diagnosed, if only the TSH tests were interpreted using accurate normal ranges. At that time, **the old TSH range (from 0.5 to 5.5) was changed to 0.3 to 3.0 by the AACE**. This means that Dr. Ridgeway's estimates of 13 million might actually involve **20 million or more people** who would find that they have some degree of thyroid problem, **if they were only TSH tested**.

- Also in 2001, the **Rotterdam studies showed that having a thyroid condition was a separate, independent risk factor for heart disease and stroke**. This study underscored the importance of a thyroid problem not only as a mild incidental illness but also as a condition that could affect and worsen other serious conditions. (Hofman)

What Do These Statistics Tell Us?

- Thyroid conditions are among the **most common** ailments today.

- In any given population, thyroid problems are epidemic.

- Those who know that they have thyroid issues represent only half of those who actually *do* have the condition.

- Thyroid problems exist in a variety of mild early forms, very difficult to detect.

- Standard screening tests reveal *severe* forms of high and low thyroid, but they are *not* sufficiently able to reveal *milder forms*.

- Millions of people suffer every day with symptoms that could be a common sign of thyroid problems. **Since most doctors are not curious about the thyroid connection,** you must be your own advocate for your best treatment.

In the late 2000s other studies began appearing, showing that **even mild forms of high and low thyroid are actually clinically significant** (see Appendix). It was then realized that **you could have** *very mild thyroid imbalance* and still have a tremendously **difficult problem** as a result of that mild medical condition.

The Many Faces of Thyroid Problems

Most people think of low thyroid as a small problem, causing a weight issue or making the person chilly or tired. This attitude, sadly, allows most thyroid problems today to remain undiagnosed and poorly treated. Now, with the work of a newly forming Coalition for Better Thyroid Care, we are moving toward a more comprehensive understanding of the poor misunderstood thyroid gland.

- **Severe forms** of thyroid disorder can cause physical collapse, hospitalization, and coma.
- **Milder forms** of the condition commonly cause fatigue, overweight, high cholesterol, high blood pressure, constipation, heart irregularity, dry hair, dry skin, dry eyes, hair thinning or hair loss, and thin, cracking, or peeling nails.
- A wide range of **female problems** can result from thyroid malfunction, including menstrual irregularity, endometriosis, infertility, recurrent miscarriage, birth defects, and terrible menopause.

Specifically, those contending with a *high thyroid* must learn to recognize the following symptoms, which can include bulging eyes; intense, staring gaze; fast pulse; irregular or skipped heartbeats; swollen, tender thyroid gland; breathlessness; feeling too hot for no reason; and nondiet-related weight loss, often with increased appetite and loose bowels.

To compound this dilemma, **any of these problems could exist alone, or mixed in with other symptoms**. The symptoms can be intermittent and mild, or they can be ongoing and severe. Thyroid problems express themselves with a tremendous variability. In many cases, this can present challenges for harried doctors who don't have the resources to spend hours interviewing their patients. Many people with thyroid problems walk out of their doctor's office with a prescription for an antidepressant. **Too many women are being misdiagnosed and undertreated for simple thyroid issues that could be easily fixed.** Thyroid imbalance, present today in epidemic proportions, commonly also causes psychological symptoms, ranging from mildly annoying behaviors to severe psychiatric disturbances. (Patrick)

Introducing the Thyroid Brain

Thyroid disease is one illness that is known to cause physical as well as mental symptoms.

> **Even mild low thyroid can cause severe physical problems and *severe mental problems*.**

These mental symptoms occur because of particular ways that the thyroid affects brain chemistry. *It is absolutely remarkable how essential the thyroid is to normal brain function.*

The brain uses thyroid differently—and more eagerly—than other tissues do. In fact, according to Ridha Arem, MD, author of *The Thyroid Solution*: "It is time for thyroid hormones to be recognized as key brain chemicals, whose actions and effects are similar in many ways to serotonin and other neuro-transmitters." (Arem)

According to Dr. Arem, an endocrinology professor and medical journal editor, **thyroid disease often remains undiagnosed for an inexcusably long time.** Dr. Arem writes, "Millions of people suffer needlessly while their doctors continue to treat thyroid dysfunction as a simple physical disorder rather than what it is: a complex blow to the body **and the mind.**"

Dr. Arem expresses concern that psychiatrists far too often are likely to come up with a psychiatric diagnosis when examining a thyroid patient. "Often, psychiatrists do not perform a detailed enough physical examination, or a complete enough panel of lab tests, that might lead them to detect physical causes for the mental symptoms."

Dr. Arem is not alone in his beliefs. A major article for *General Hospital Psychiatry* describes the following study (Kathol):

> In a group of hyperthyroid patients seen by psychiatrists, almost half were diagnosed with depression, or anxiety disorder. These patients did not have anxiety or depression however; what they had were the *mental symptoms* of hyperthyroidism.

If trained psychiatrists are making this misdiagnosis, just imagine how many general practitioners, internists, busy clinic doctors, and urgent care doctors might make this same kind of mistake.

- The issue is that the doctor does not see that an underlying thyroid condition can explain the psychiatric symptoms in full.
- Also unacknowledged is the possibility that simple thyroid treatment might relieve these symptoms rather quickly and effectively.

Faced with this monumental challenge, modern medicine has taken an unfortunately casual stance. The condition is checked for, but often not that carefully. The condition is sometimes treated, but not that vigorously. Health workers educate the public, but for the most part not that effectively. The epidemic is being addressed, but not very well.

We have a growing epidemic in full progress. It is an epidemic affecting metabolism and brain function. Large numbers of people are involved.

Simultaneously, we are seeing a skyrocketing incidence of diabetes and obesity in both adults and children. There is ample evidence that large amounts of these other epidemics are simply spin-offs of the epidemic of thyroid hormone malfunction.

If you are wondering what could possibly be causing such widespread thyroid disruption, you won't have to look very far. It turns out that the last 40 years have witnessed a massive increase in the amount of hormone-disrupting synthetic chemicals finding their way into our air, food, and water.

This toxic pollution, originally addressed by Rachel Carson in her 1962 groundbreaking book *Silent Spring,* is a major culprit. (Carson) By the 1980s even more conclusive evidence was showing that **hormonally active synthetic waste chemicals were indeed causing a huge amount of health disruption**. The most sensitive and highly susceptible of human tissues turned out to be the thyroid gland.

In the mid-1990s a monumental collection of this evidence was published in a book called *Our Stolen Future*. (Colborn) In the late 1990s a remarkable follow-up volume by Sheldon Krimsky was called *Hormonal Chaos*. The environmental-endocrine story was now moving from the status of a theory to the reality of another inconvenient truth. (Krimsky)

What is at stake here is the health of our nation, and our world.

What is at stake is the **quality of life for many millions of people**. Since low thyroid can contribute to the worsening of other conditions, such as high blood pressure and cholesterol, it is also likely that thyroid problems may be to blame for the early demise of some people.

A New Role for Nurses

If doctors have been constrained by managed care, then perhaps nurses could become more proactive to help millions suffering. Nurses, who see people in hospitals and clinics, could be on the forefront of early thyroid diagnosis and treatment, simply by ensuring that supposedly "well" people could receive proper evaluation for their hidden thyroid conditions *before* they become severely ill.

Nurses can also ensure that more patients in hospitals and clinical settings receive adequate testing if they show suspicious symptoms. It is a simple matter to add thyroid testing to any other blood panel.

Thousands of other practitioners can also become more informed, including counselors and therapists, dieticians and nutritionists, respiratory therapists, physical therapists, and body workers. These caregivers could be more active in directing their clients to those doctors or nurse practitioners who demonstrate enough curiosity to make sure their patients receive proper diagnosis and care for underlying thyroid disorders. With a higher index of suspicion, more thyroid conditions could be diagnosed and well treated.

New Fixes for Chronic Conditions

What if a significant amount of mood and behavior could be improved with better thyroid balance? Scientists and researchers have long known it is possible—yet standard health care has displayed a monumental lack of curiosity in considering this option.

Research has already demonstrated the beneficial mental health results from using nature-made products, such as St. John's wort and SAM-e. Yet insurance companies continue to pay enormous amounts of money only for pharmaceuticals, money they charge to health consumers as high premiums.

How can the frontiers of standard medicine possibly improve using the same tired, old thinking?

Modern medical dogma dictates that doctors treat every patient with a diagnosed condition by using only the remedy generally accepted as specific for that condition, regardless of the unique needs of the person treated. In our present culture, chronic conditions have become the Achilles' heel of our fast-paced society.

We can do better than this. Not only do we present a program here for healing the millions of thyroid-related psychological situations, but we also present an improved model for approaching chronic illness.

In this book, we suggest a new model for many chronic conditions now plaguing our society, especially for mental illness and emotional imbalances.

Most thyroid issues are autoimmune related, as are many of the most common illnesses of our time. We contend that many debilitating and chronic conditions can be improved, using the same perspective we present here for thyroid conditions.

You might be saying, "Listen, symptom-relieving prescription medicine, when it does work, is effective and quick." We would agree with you. Karilee thanks her lucky stars—and the scientists—for having Imitrex available during her migraine years. But does this solve the entire problem? No, it serves only to temporarily relieve the person's symptoms.

What it *will not* do is improve the root cause of problems.

It does not fully correct the hormonal brain chemistry imbalance.

Meet the Thyroid Dilemma

To keep medical practice profitable, doctors have been squeezed into seeing more people per hour.

> **In a shortened appointment time, there simply is not adequate time to take a detailed enough history and give a thorough physical exam to get to the bottom of a hormonal or physical cause of psychological behaviors.**

It is barely enough time to suggest to the patient a symptom-relieving psychiatric drug and then write a prescription for it.

While this model of practice may help people with colds and flu, **it is not an appropriate model for people with lifelong thyroid-caused psychological challenges that have never been properly addressed.** We propose a more comprehensive model, with a program that ensures adequate ongoing support until the thyroid dilemma is fully reversed.

> **Find a practitioner who can take the time to sort out your possible thyroid issues.**

Challenges We Face, Together

The **thyroid situation presents a perfect microcosm** for everything that is wrong in our current medical system. Specialists are often so focused on their tiny corner of the human body that a patient is only viewed from that one perspective at a time, when what is ailing him or her may actually be interwoven among a variety of related body systems.

Our hormonal system interacts with our nervous system, for example, carrying information that regulates the brain and nerves. In turn, the brain constantly sends chemical and electrical messages to regulate the hormonal system. These complex interactions are crucial, a fascinating part of our biochemical dance, from conception until death.

Learning to decipher these messages and to correct an imbalanced biochemistry is one of the greatest challenges and opportunities of our lives.

> **The revolution in psychiatric medication transforming the mental health landscape cannot by itself cure the mental ills of those we love.**

Many times our uncomfortable emotional states, such as anxiety, agitation, depression, rage, and others, stem from a hormonal source. If you come from a hormonally challenged family, you could go through your entire lifetime feeling unable to control your own behavior. You may feel ashamed, hiding it as best you can, feeling hopeless that you may ever be able to gain control of yourself.

Karilee's Story

In my younger life, anger was my constant companion. Perhaps I was born this way; certainly I inherited some of this from my mother, her father, his parents, and so it goes. There was plenty of anger to go around in our household.

I hated being yelled at and hit repeatedly as a child. I swore that I would never do this to my own children. Yet, when Shauna was only a baby, our babysitter kept suggesting I stop yelling at the baby; exhausted, I didn't even realize I had been.

Things got worse when we had our second daughter. The older child, only 2 years old, was waking in the middle of the night screaming in terror, having bad dreams, waking the baby, causing us all to lose crucial hours of sleep.

After months of this, I was beyond desperate. I recall one day starting to push my elder child's face into the rug, being totally out of control, and suddenly awakening as if from a bad dream.

I saw in my own behavior a reflection of my mother and all those before her who were out of control. Perhaps it was my innate guidance that stopped me from the repetition compulsion pattern that was unconsciously ingrained within me on some very deep level.

It was as if I stepped back and could see what I was doing, and I was appalled. Fortunately, our babysitting team encouraged me to attend co-counseling classes in our town.

There was a Birth Center then (thank you, Denny Ferry, wherever you are, magical woman) helping parents of young kids to get together, hear each other's stories, and learn new coping tools. I learned to rage at the bed (not my child), to use a foam bat to beat the crap out of pillows, to scream at the top of my lungs when I needed to, and to gain enough control to make sure I did *not* hit my children ever.

(continued)

Another critical tool was a careful check of my hormones. Tests revealed that the previously "healed" thyroid problem of my early twenties had come back, likely triggered by the recent birth. Based on testing, I went back on thyroid medicine and felt much calmer and more in control.

I practiced these coping tools on and off for years; they saved our lives. I shared this work over time, helping my patients learn to let go of their anger and fear, their sadness and disappointment. I learned through teaching, as we often do, eventually finding new ways to rebalance my own biochemical makeup, which has contributed to greater serenity and success in my emotional life.

I consider myself quite fortunate to have lived in a time when self-exploration and thyroid hormone testing were encouraged. I have been able to learn tools of communication and biochemical assessment, which older generations were not given. All of these have helped my generation to move forward. I hope to make a small contribution toward that evolution through the sharing of these stories.

When the Engine Is Broken, the Car Doesn't Work

Think of the thyroid as the engine and energy regulator for everything else in your body. The thyroid can be viewed as a metaphor in many ways. In her own personal explorations, it became clear to Karilee that the thyroid "lives" between the head and heart, perhaps helping these seemingly opposite parts of our selves to stay connected. It can be viewed as a "mystical mediator," directing traffic, working closely with other glands in a biochemical fishbowl from which our actions are spawned.

The thyroid gland is housed in the throat. According to the ancient Hindu philosophy, this is in the fifth energy center (*chakra* in Sanskrit), related to self-expression and communication. It is a center related to *speaking one's truth*. On our long journey, we have come to believe that the thyroid is related to our hearts, minds, and communications.

Our nervous system is partially regulated by the thyroid. We can often improve agitation, anxiety, depression, anger, and irritability, all by working directly with the thyroid.

And while we are confident that you can sense the magical role the thyroid plays in our physical and emotional lives, we also hope you can see how this discussion could apply to *chronic conditions in general*. For all these reasons, we consider the thyroid to be a helpful metaphor.

When something is wrong with your engine, everything else is affected. In our years of practice, we have seen thousands of people, perhaps three-fourths women and one-fourth men, trudge into our office feeling unhealthy. They may have one symptom, sometimes several symptoms, occasionally even a long list of symptoms. They may have been experiencing these problems for years, often without adequate help. Some had even asked for thyroid care, all to no avail.

In addition, they often feel angry, discouraged, and discounted. All this remains on top of their original mental symptoms, which they partially attribute to feeling discouraged for years and years and being physically sick for so long. When medical professionals listen to them at all, it is usually to prescribe an antidepressant, as if the whole problem is "all in their head."

For many of them, the problem is really "all in their neck." Frequently, after years of unsuccessful intervention, a high percentage of these multisystem sufferers get largely or completely better, with simple thyroid treatment. Receiving the right dose of the right medicine can reverse sluggish function in many aspects of their lives.

More discouraging, however, is when some of these same people come to see us having been properly diagnosed, but only *partially treated* for the underlying thyroid problem. All too frequently, they report to us the sad result wherein physical ailments have subsided, but the mental and emotional symptoms remain.

The Thyroid-Mind Connection

It is this latter group to which we have paid closest attention in recent years.

Our clinical experience has proven to us that aggressively pursuing optimal thyroid treatment has resulted in more complete psychological healing.

Freddy's Story

Freddy Barrett was a child prodigy until age 14, when it all changed. He had always been the smartest kid in his class, exceedingly gifted at math and physics. Surprisingly, he combined brain and brawn, being successfully competitive at junior high track and field.

Then, in the middle of eighth grade, he started losing his edge and interest in sports. His grades took a nosedive as well. The previously dependable drive and ambition seemed to fade away. Even his well-known sense of humor had disappeared. He had plenty of physical strength and energy, but no interest in using it.

For Freddy, everything was now either "boring" or "too much trouble." He grew grouchy and irritable with friends and family alike.

No, he had not gotten into drugs. Definitely not. In his case, it seemed a simple teen depression, but neither psychotherapy nor medication yielded any benefit. When encouraged by teachers or school counselors to build on his prior success, his response was always: "Nah, I'm not interested in that anymore." This gradually became "High school is such bull****; just leave me alone."

His parents did no such thing. Instead, they insisted that the current psychiatrist send the now-18-year-old dropout to our Preventive Medicine Center for hormone evaluation. All tests were

Men Do Too Have Thyroid Conditions!

There are several key takeaways from the story above. First, Freddy is obviously male. If you are a man reading this book, understand that this is *not just a woman's disease*—it could easily happen to you. If you are a woman, realize that the men in your life could easily be affected, maybe with similar lack of positive lab tests. Thus, while mostly women get this condition, men *do* get it. And men often have different symptoms.

Men tend more toward apathy, depression, and listlessness when they have a thyroid condition.

They can gain weight, but do not always. Sometimes, amazingly, their normal, except for borderline low thyroid. The parents, knowing of a thyroid family history, conferred with their son and agreed to initiate a trial of thyroid treatment.

"After all," the mom said, "what harm could a mild dose of thyroid do?" Once adjusted to the proper level of medicine, Fred's downward behavior spiral began making a turnaround. Within weeks, his mood and energy noticeably improved. After another month, he seemed much more like his old self.

Retesting showed that the previously modest but "high normal" levels of thyroid antibodies were now completely gone. In addition, his body temperature had returned from slightly below normal to now fully normal. Without any prodding, he got back into his jogging routine each morning and thus began to feel even better.

Now, Fred is in college, fully recovered, and once again happily at the top of his class. His experience illustrates the profound effects that even borderline low thyroid can have on purely mental/emotional realms. Except for slightly low body temperature, he never had physical signs of low thyroid. He never even had the abnormal blood tests of low thyroid. What he did have, however, was **low thyroid**.

Once his thyroid was treated, he got his life back. Sadly, he missed the best of his high school years. Happily, he now has a long productive life ahead of him.

only physical symptom is high cholesterol! At times there are no physical symptoms, just a vague malaise, feeling off your usual pace.

In a more severe form, there can be deep depression, severe irritability, and an unexpected tendency toward violent or addictive behavior. Even though most thyroid sufferers are women, there are still millions of men who are liable to be dealing with low thyroid and not know it.

A trial of thyroid hormone can help to diagnose the condition as well as help to fix it.

The second intriguing aspect of the Freddy story is that even though the tests did not show a definite diagnosis, a trial of thyroid medicine was nevertheless a good idea.

Frequently, a medicine trial can be extremely useful for evalua-tion. This is especially true given the current sad state of thyroid testing. We address this topic fully in Chapter 9. Even as Freddy's parents agreed, "If it doesn't work, at least we tried, and no harm done." We want to be very clear about this:

> A trial of thyroid medicine in a dose appropriate to the person's age, height, and weight is *not* risky.

It is a rather benign medical intervention, having no effect whatsoever if the person's thyroid status was normal to begin with. On the other hand, if a person's thyroid status was not normal originally, then the results are frequently quite helpful.

A trial of thyroid medicine is also useful diagnostically, to help rule in or rule out abnormal cortisol status. The reason for this is that taking thyroid when the person has low cortisol levels results in a benign wors-ening of the low cortisol symptoms; feeling worse tells us more about your case.

Standard blood testing is only adequate to rule in or rule out Cushing's or Addison's disease, the very extremes of high and low corti-sol levels. What we are talking about here is **mild cortisol imbalance**, one that can be revealed by a mildly adverse response to a thyroid medicine trial.

Overcoming a Current Failure of Modern Medicine

As a doctor, nurse, and acupuncturist, we do not believe that our focus here should be to tackle all the shortcomings of our current health deliv-ery system. Instead, there is one easy fix that we are highly qualified to recommend. It is actually very easy and could be readily implemented. **Fix the thyroid!**

We feel it is critical that practicing medical doctors, nurse practitio-ners, physician assistants, and other general care providers become more aware of this important connection. As observers and caregivers, they have the ability to make a huge difference in the lives of many of their patients.

One Simple Solution: Fix the Thyroid First!

Millions of people are being misdiagnosed, and undertreated, especially when it comes to thyroid care.

If you or someone you love is living with depression, do the right thing—even if your current doctor hasn't—*get a full thyroid evaluation*. If you find results showing that you even possibly could have a thyroid problem (if your results are near the high or low end of the scale), consider starting on some thyroid-boosting maneuvers. (See Chapters 4 through 8 for specific suggestions.) If they help you, continue them and add more over time.

Psycho-pharmaceutical drugs are often extremely costly and can have significant side effects. While the "quick fix" is the easy route, it may not be the best one for you or your loved ones for the long haul. Depression is a sluggishness of the brain chemicals causing mood challenges.

Why not first boost the brain, and see if you feel better?

Sometimes the simple wisdom is best. Use common sense and take steps today to help yourself or someone you care about. Thyroid care is so much less expensive than the alternatives; *check your thyroid well.*

The following chapters will walk you through a step-by-step process to help you determine whether your thyroid could be causing your mental or emotional symptoms. We look forward to helping you determine if you could be thyroid challenged, and how that might be affecting your personal brain function. You will also be given specific directions about how to begin to improve your thyroid-related symptoms.

We wish you good traveling on an exciting and rewarding journey.

Complementary Healing for Your Best Results

By Georjana Shames, LAc

At the root of Acupuncture practice is an integrative philosophy in which mind and body are closely connected at all times.

Acupuncture practice treats both the emotional content of one's life and physical symptoms that arise in illness.

Those of us who grew up in the contemporary Western world sometimes find it difficult to conceptualize what we mean when we talk about a patient who has mental symptoms that arise from a physical cause—for example, anxiety that stems from a thyroid imbalance.

To a conventional allopathic physician, a patient might appear to have two separate constellations of symptoms: symptoms that arise from a mental cause and symptoms that arise in a physical way. For example, consider a menopausal woman who presents at the clinic with pain and soreness of the lower back, afternoon fever, feeling of heat, insomnia, dry throat especially at night, irritation, and mental restlessness.

To the allopathic practitioner, it appears she has some physical symptoms and some mental symptoms. The physical soreness of the back and hot flashes are purely **physical**. From a separate perspective, she has **mental** symptoms like mental restlessness, difficulty calming the mind, and a feeling of being uncomfortable and irritated.

Now this same woman could present at an acupuncturist's office; the acupuncturist would perceive these symptoms in a holistic way by virtue of the philosophy of Chinese Medicine.

The acupuncturist would look at this same constellation of symptoms and see that the mental symptoms and the physical symptoms stem from the same imbalance, arising from the same source.

To understand what we mean when we describe a source of an imbalance, let us first talk briefly about Acupuncture theory as it pertains to the various internal meridians.

Each of the 14 main meridians in the human body has a specific function and various constellations of symptoms that arise when it is out of balance.

When we talk about the **Lung Meridian**, for example, we are not describing the physical lung within the chest cavity, but rather an energetic pathway that corresponds to the function of what the Lung Meridian is responsible for in Acupuncture theory. The Lung Meridian is responsible for drawing heavenly air into the human body, creating what we call Qi, or **fuel that the body runs on**.

MORE EXAMPLES OF MERIDIAN THEORY

- The **Large Intestine Meridian**, again, is not a physical organ but is a representation of the function of the body's system of **elimination**.

- The **Stomach Meridian** is integral to the **metabolism**, as is the **Spleen Meridian**, which is very important to extracting the benefits of nutrition from what you eat.

- The **Heart Meridian** very closely corresponds to the **emotional** content of our lives.

- It is said in Acupuncture theory: *"The Heart houses the Mind."*

- We can tell immediately that the Heart Meridian is closely connected to any kind of mental restlessness, worry, anxiety, or depression.

- Another very important aspect of this meridian is that *"The Heart governs the Blood"*—not necessarily the physical blood that pumps through your veins, but rather a function of Blood in Chinese Medicine, which is to nourish the organs and muscles.

- When it comes to mental health in Acupuncture theory, the Blood and the Yin are both closely connected to the emotions, since the Yin is very calming, relaxing energy and the Blood is nourishing energy.

If we take the metaphor of a car being akin to the human body, Yin would be the coolant for the car's engine, Blood would be the oil nourishing all the mechanical connections, and Yang would be the gasoline fueling the car.

It is said in Acupuncture theory that Blood and Yin are the residence of the Mind. If these are abundant, the person will feel mentally happy and vital. If Blood and Yin are deficient, the Mind will suffer, and the person will feel depressed and lack vitality.

We have so far talked a bit about the functions of the Lung Meridian, Large Intestine Meridian, Stomach Meridian, Spleen Meridian, and Heart Meridian. Now let us turn our attention to briefly covering the others.

The **Small Intestine Meridian** has a very fascinating function to play when it comes to mental health. It is said that the Small Intestine Meridian is responsible for *"separating pure from impure."* A person who is deeply affected by emotional or mental factors has *difficulty separating priorities from irrelevancies.* This is a crucial ability for a healthy life, learning to separate for oneself who should be an influence on your life and whom you should steer clear of.

The **Bladder Meridian** illustrates an excellent example of the mind-body connection, which works from the Western perspective as well as the Chinese perspective. When we are suddenly distressed from fear, our mental anxiety causes the Bladder Meridian to become instantly weakened; the Kidney and Bladder Meridians cannot hold the Qi. (In plain words, when we are shocked into acute mental fright, we may suddenly pee. This is an example of a mind-body connection at its most visceral.)

The **Kidney Meridian** is the root of the body's energy, and it often relates to *fear*. There is an aspect of the Kidney Meridian that is closely tied to our survival. When we become afraid for our health, afraid for our business, afraid for our finances, we often experience this as a threat to our very survival (even when unwarranted).

As you have gathered thus far in this book, mild hormone imbalances generally do not kill anyone, but they can make you wish you were dead— or make you feel like you are living only half your life. This strikes to the heart of our very survival instinct.

Speaking of strikes to the heart, the **Pericardium Meridian** is known as the "Heart Protector" in Chinese Medicine, akin to the Emperor's bodyguard. The **Liver Meridian** is considered the seat of the emotions in Chinese Medicine.

Now we can see a connection between the Heart Meridian (which houses the Mind) and Liver Meridian (responsible for the smooth flow of emotions).

Depression is essentially an example of a stagnation of the emotions caused by obstruction of the smooth flow of the Liver Meridian.

The **Liver** relates to **anger**, as does the **Gallbladder Meridian**; thus there is a connection in Acupuncture theory between pent-up emotions— such as anger, frustration, rage—and the Liver Meridian and Gallbladder Meridian.

The final two pathways, the **Governing Meridian** and the **Conception Meridian**, are closely linked to the Kidney Meridian. They are used in clinical practice to deeply affect the patient's energy at a profound level.

AN INTEGRATIVE PERSPECTIVE

Now that you know a bit about the various meridians in Acupuncture theory, let us go back to the menopausal woman presenting with symptoms that appear to arise from two different sources (a mental source and a physical source) but, in fact, are arising from the same imbalance. Her actual imbalance is a lack of Kidney Yin, the cooling energy, which then gave rise to Heart Heat, which involves mental restlessness, emotional edginess, and difficulty in calming oneself.

Here we have a pattern identification in Acupuncture perspective that accounts for the entire constellation of symptoms: a deficiency in the Kidney can cause a sore back, pain in the joints, and dry throat at night, and the Heart Heat accounts for her mental restlessness, her edginess, all of the mental and emotional symptoms the patient is experiencing.

When we see from an Acupuncture perspective that one imbalance can cause both physical and mental symptoms, we know that the wisest course of action is to *treat both* simultaneously. Nourishing her Kidney Yin will help soothe the Heart Heat; in this way we can treat both the person's mental anguish *and* her physical discomforts. (Maciocia)

An acupuncturist would be remiss if she did not treat both aspects; in this view, they are so closely interconnected that they simply cannot be separated. Over time one causes the other. Mental anguish creates physical symptoms, and physical symptoms result in mental stress. Over time a lack of cooling Kidney Yin energy causes the Heart Meridian to be agitated by Heat, or conversely Heart Heat burns out Kidney Yin.

Either way, ultimately the patient is struggling with both mental and physical imbalances. Fortunately, the great news is that both aspects can benefit from acupuncture treatment.

THE BOTTOM LINE

- Thyroid imbalance is surprisingly one of the most common of all medical conditions.
- Thyroid problems also become more common as we age.
- Standard screening tests reveal **severe forms** of high and low thyroid but are **not** sufficiently able to reveal **milder forms**.
- You could have *very mild thyroid imbalance,* yet still have a **difficult problem** as a result of that mild medical condition.
- The **delicate hormonal balance that keeps us focused and sensible** has been largely lost, replaced by a hormonal imbalance causing many to act strangely without knowing why.
- Too many women are being misdiagnosed, and undertreated for simple thyroid issues that could be easily fixed.
- **Thyroid imbalance**, present today in epidemic proportions, **commonly causes psychological symptoms** ranging from annoying behaviors to severe psychiatric disturbances.

- *Even **mild** low thyroid* can cause *severe physical problems* and severe mental problems as well.
- Thyroid is absolutely *essential* for normal brain function.
- The last 40 years have witnessed a massive increase in the amount of hormone-disrupting synthetic chemicals finding their way into our air, food, and water.

RECOMMENDED ACTION PLAN

- Find a practitioner who can take time to sort out your possible thyroid issues.
- **Our nervous system is partially regulated by thyroid.** We can improve our agitation, anxiety, depression, anger, and irritability, all by working directly with the thyroid.
- **Puberty, childbirth, and menopause** are well-known triggers that often cause years of thyroid problems for predisposed people.
- Accidents, illness, surgery, bereavement, fear, major sleep loss, or prolonged overwork also can contribute to thyroid problems.
- Men tend more toward apathy, depression, and listlessness when they do have a thyroid condition.
- A trial of thyroid hormone can help to diagnose the condition as well as help to fix it.
- Thyroid problems at times cause mental symptoms that can occur without any accompanying physical symptoms.
- Acupuncture practice treats both the *emotional* content of one's life and the *physical symptoms* that arise in illness.
- Begin to see beyond the artificial distinction of mind and body as separate.

2

Thyroid Imbalance Often Causes Mental Imbalance

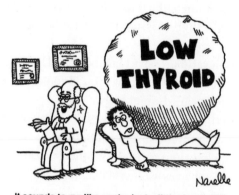

It sounds to me like you're just a little depressed.

If we tell you about the wild women in our families of origin, will you try not to think less of us as health professionals? What if we told you that emotional imbalances were commonplace in our birth families?

The reality is that had our families been perfectly "normal," we would most likely never have written this book. The similarities in our origins may be responsible for our coming together and understanding each other through 30 years of marriage. These common emotional patterns from our early lives have also brought havoc into our marriage at various times.

The complexity of biochemistry in the women in our families has made it imperative that we try to ameliorate these hormonal issues—for our patients as well as for the sake of our unborn grandchildren.

We feel at times like medical missionaries, traveling through the annals of medicine, guided by the tender patience of our patients, for whom this book is written. Our quest is to find the "holy grail," the chalice that will quench the thirst of those suffering with emotional dysfunctions related to thyroid imbalance.

We will not rest until more of you are feeling better, enjoying your lives.

We have come to know this mental anguish through our own personal stories, and through those who have sought hormonal balance in our medical office practice. We have dedicated our time and resources to developing new ways to empower you and your loved ones to fix these problems and learn to enjoy your lives more each day.

Karilee's diagnosis came at age 20, when she became desperately ill while studying in Spain. Recalling her uncomfortable adolescence, she now feels certain she was struggling with thyroid issues long before the crisis that allowed her to get diagnosed.

She was overweight, with low-level depressive tendencies and low self-esteem. It turns out that thyroid problems often show around adolescence and—when fixed—can improve those years dramatically.

Reflecting back on our respective family trees, we wonder if any of the women in our families did *not* have a thyroid problem. Both of Karilee's grandmothers were diagnosed with low thyroid. Rich's mother was on thyroid medicine ever since he can remember, as was her sister, his aunt. Today most of Karilee's siblings take thyroid medication.

Is it environment or heredity? This question often arises when pursuing causal aspects of health and behavior. Though they cannot be separated completely, we do know that thyroid conditions are highly inherited.

Most important, however, we do know now that when mental symptoms are present, thyroid *must* be considered.

Explorations in the Thyroid-Mind Connection

As we have expanded our explorations of the growing thyroid epidemic, we have seen a strong tendency for people with thyroid problems to become depressed or agitated. More and more of our patients complain of depression, or mood or behavior challenges.

We believe the growing epidemic of low thyroid closely mirrors the growing epidemic of psychological impairment we are witnessing in today's violent culture.

While various unsatisfying explanations have been proposed regarding this mounting societal burden of psychological illness, scientists are rapidly coming to agreement that *one major cause* of the mounting epidemic of thyroid dysfunction is largely due to the proliferation of chemical pollution in the air, food, and water. Many of these chemicals are hormone disrupters, altering proper thyroid balance.

One troublesome result of this massive thyroid problem is that we now have a society filled with people behaving strangely; many are seemingly exaggerated in their previous behaviors, showing rampant imbalances, experiencing annoyances ranging from mild anxiety to xenophobia (fear of strangers).

These *physically caused mental symptoms* have been noted from the earliest medical literature, a great metaphor being the mythical story of Nero fiddling while Rome burned. This is considered an example of a very common dementia of the time, diagnosed centuries later through bone examinations as lead poisoning, which came from the lead-lined Roman aqueducts and lead cooking utensils.

Lead poisoning causes mental disturbances.

Today we do not have lead-lined aqueducts, but we *do* have significant amounts of hormone-disrupting synthetic chemical pollution and **hormone-disrupting heavy metal contamination**, including fluoridation products contaminated with lead and mercury that are being put in our waters.

Today most people affected by the current epidemic are taking antidepressants or other mental medications in their attempts to feel better. **While these drugs may offer tentative relief, they do not address the root cause.**

What's at Stake?

The proliferation of mental imbalances causes problems for individuals, marriages, families, friends, and work relationships. These problems can eventually contribute to larger community and societal issues. Problems range from low sex drive to seasonal affective disorder, retardation, and autism—which are known to have strong thyroid connections.

The brain and its emotional responses are more affected by thyroid than are other bodily tissues.

There is a positive note, however:

A great deal of this suffering can be remedied readily and inexpensively.

We start by addressing two glaring facts:

1. The current testing for ruling out the thyroid (especially for mental problems) is woefully inadequate.

2. Even if thyroid hormone levels are well tested and shown to be normal, **you could still have thyroid-related mental/ behavioral challenges** because of an interference in your nervous system by thyroid antibodies.

A Growing Epidemic

Our country is experiencing a mushrooming epidemic of thyroid malfunction, mirroring a parallel epidemic of mood and behavior disorders. Many researchers believe there is a causal relationship, that the mounting incidence of thyroid imbalance is, in part, directly responsible for the mounting incidence of psychological illness.

Most people would be surprised to learn how very often thyroid problems can cause mental symptoms. Of the 40 million Americans with thyroid problems, almost all have some degree of mental symptoms along with physical ones. The mental symptoms include difficulty with calculation or remembering names, words on the tip of the tongue but not expressed easily, or actual difficulty with focus and planning. Psychological symptoms range from anxiety, irritability, annoyances with everyday life, and mild sadness to severe and profound depression, mood swings that become more common and exaggerated, unusual and new fears, and even phobias and panic, as well as outright psychosis. Many people, women especially, experience unpleasant emotions.

Katie's Story

At the age of 27, Katie Schwartz, a comedy writer, was on the precipice of a successful career. She was at the pinnacle of health, weighing 135 pounds, running 6 miles a day, with a steady mood and clear head, and maintaining a vegetarian diet. Life with her canine son, Louie, was amazingly good.

Over the next 5 years, she began to exhibit increasingly severe psychiatric symptoms—moodiness, irritability, forgetfulness, paranoia, anxiety, and a bit of bipolar disorder—as well as physical symptoms. Though perplexed by this, she chalked it up to stress, as she was working 70 hours a week.

As she continued to see her MD, he reported that her white blood cell count was elevating up to 25,000 (normal is 5,000 to 6,000). He assured her this was no cause for concern.

Then Katie began gaining weight. She still did not have a diagnosis, or know that this was thyroid related. Physical symptoms that she experienced included fierce diarrhea, rapid heart rate, profuse sweating, hand tremors, muscle weakness in all extremities, and thyroid storms (sudden excessive secretion of thyroid hormone from the irritated gland). Her inability to breathe forced her to stop running.

One day, she woke up with swollen eyelids. Thinking this was precipitated by her chronic insomnia, she didn't give it a second thought—until 2 weeks later, when she went from having 20/20 vision to viewing everything through a "murky aquarium."

Dozens of specialists eager to dispense their "scrip-tails" (cocktails of prescription medicine) that they were sure would cure what they couldn't diagnose only served to exacerbate her symptoms, rendering her a semi-reclusive mess (her words).

Incapable of taking meetings, concentrating, or achieving deadlines; delirious; severely depressed; extremely paranoid; and experiencing odd menstrual cycles, crazy rashes, hair loss, and a host of other couldn't-connect-the-dots symptoms, Katie was in a state of severe physical and mental trauma.

In one appointment with Jules Stein Eye Institute for her eyes, she was given a possible diagnosis, "Graves' eye disease," and a referral to an endocrinologist. Without knowing what an endocrinologist was, much less what they did, her mother dragged her daughter to the doctor.

(continued)

Katie learned that one of the specialists she'd seen previously had tested her thyroid but didn't tell her—he had just told her everything was *normal*. Perhaps he did not understand the meaning of her results.

He felt her neck; she asked why. He matter-of-factly stated: "That's where your thyroid is." She had no idea what a thyroid was or did. Without much explanation, he put her on a drug, Tapazole. For whatever reason, she had a severe, unusual adverse reaction to it.

Within 12 months, she became 100% thyroid psychotic and borderline thyro-toxic. Her mother and sister staged an intervention to literally save her life. She was given a radioactive iodine (RAI) treatment to destroy the overactive thyroid gland. Sadly, they told her she had no other option.

She later found out that she would have been in a coma or died within a few weeks.

Six weeks post-treatment, she felt like she had woken up from a coma and a hurricane, combined. She didn't recognize herself. She had very few memories of what had happened during her psychoses.

She now feels that had her mother and sister not been so brave, she wouldn't be here today. She is still deeply saddened by the heartache she caused her mother and sister, two of the greatest loves of her life.

Though mistreatment persisted by the next five endocrinologists over the course of 5 years (her words), she continues finding her way back to herself. She has learned that this disease is a process. She now has a wonderful integrative specialist and psychiatrist.

We are pleased to tell you that Katie is now back to being a joyful functioning person. Based on her own experiences, she is working with others in the Coalition for Better Thyroid Care, to help make sure this does not happen to you. Her writing career is flourishing once again, and she is also the founder of Dear Thyroid (www.DearThyroid .org), seeking to rebrand the face of thyroid disease and offer support, awareness, and education. Thyroid patients write and submit love and hate letters to their thyroids, among other literary things. Dear Thyroid has ongoing columns about various thyroid diseases and cancers, as well as aggressive outreach, awareness, and support programs, both online and offline. What makes Dear Thyroid unique is that 99% of the site is written by and for thyroid patients.

After speaking with thousands of thyroid patients, Katie feels that thyroid diseases are *not* taken seriously enough. The exorbitant expense of treatment, paired with the gross negligence that commonly occurs with thyroid patients, is unconscionable. She now feels that her case is not rare, which is terrifying to her. Her hope is to be part of the movement that seeks change for thyroid patients.

Brain Drives Mind;
Thyroid Drives Brain

As with any of our bodily organs, the brain requires nutrients and energy to function well. The brain, in fact, uses more energy in the form of glucose and oxygen than does any other organ. Though only about 3 pounds in weight, the brain utilizes as much as one-fourth of the body's energy output, in terms of oxygen consumption and glucose burning.

The brain, therefore, is more dependent on proper energy metabolism than is any other organ.

The thyroid controls the energy for the body and, hence, for the brain. If thyroid is too high or too low, the brain suffers accordingly. Proper brain function involves a delicate balance of many billions of neurons and their associated cells, each doing exactly what they are supposed to do at exactly the right time.

If thyroid function is askew, this crucial timing can be off. Sluggish brain function can result in sluggish thinking, possibly even depression. The actual physiological mechanisms for many of these occurrences have been studied and documented. (See Notes and References and the section "Further Reading" in Resources, both in the back of this book.)

Changes in thyroid balance can affect the amount of blood circulating through and nourishing the brain.

- A decrease in the level of thyroid hormone can result in diminished numbers and activity of mitochondria, powerhouses of the cell that supply energy for cell function.
- In addition, changes in thyroid hormone levels result in changes of the reading of the DNA genetic code and, ultimately, in the transcription of that code into cellular activity. (Dratman)

Therefore, **too much or too little thyroid hormone can result in profound changes in brain function**, often quite specific for the individual. With a similar amount of thyroid dysfunction, some have memory loss, while others may experience anxiety. Some might get depressed, while others may have increased cravings. Many will find that their sleep is affected. (Joffe)

Conditions as diverse as low sex drive and retardation are known to have strong thyroid connections. It is certainly well known that babies born to mothers critically low in thyroid hormone can be born with mental retardation.

This one small gland can be the root cause of a great many psychological symptoms. Some people with thyroid imbalance will have a tendency to become more violent, while others become docile and despondent.

Medical Progress: Blending Old and New

A quick review of the various symptoms caused by thyroid imbalance in any medical textbook will reveal, amid the "physical" symptoms, many "mental" symptoms. The list includes depression; anxiety; mood swings; panic; phobia; problems with memory, focus, and concentration; and sleep problems. Hallucinations, paranoia, schizophrenia, bipolar disorder (manic depression), postpartum psychosis, confusion, and dementia have also been attributed, in some individuals, to the physical abnormality of thyroid hormone alone.

Mental symptoms can exist *in addition to* the well-known physical symptoms, or instead of any physical symptoms.

> **Thyroid's mental symptoms can coexist with thyroid's physical symptoms in one person. You can also have thyroid's mental symptoms without experiencing the physical symptoms.**

This missed diagnosis represents an extremely common abnormality that could perhaps build a bridge of understanding between the current epidemic of *thyroid problems* that we have in our society, and our current epidemic of *depression and anxiety*. It can only help to view these two seemingly separate issues of body and mind as not so separate after all.

What does this mental and physical mix of medical symptoms actually look like in real life?

How Thyroid May Affect Your Mental Health

- If you feel mildly **nervous, anxious, agitated,** irritable, angry, enraged, depressed, or otherwise behaviorally challenged, it may be your thyroid.

- If you have a definite psychological diagnosis, **but only indefinite improvement with treatment**, it could well be your thyroid.

- If you have been fortunate enough to receive thyroid treatment, but unfortunate enough for **the mental symptoms to be persistent**, it could still be your thyroid. (Hall)

- If you have a long, **convoluted history of family** with thyroid or autoimmune problems, you could soon join the ranks.

- If thyroid is your issue, and if you can get your thyroid gland back in balance, you may receive one of life's greatest gifts—improved mental well-being.

Once again, here are categories of people that need better care:

ARE YOU UNDIAGNOSED?

- You may have been told that you do not have a thyroid problem based solely on blood testing, often using *only* the overrated TSH test.

- Or worse, you *may never have been given any thyroid testing* at all. People in this category believe they do not have a thyroid problem, but they certainly could—and a great many do.

ARE YOU MISDIAGNOSED?

- You may have been diagnosed with depression, anxiety disorder, or attention deficit disorder.

- You may even be receiving treatment for this condition, which may be helping somewhat.

- Nevertheless, the treatment may not be addressing the root cause, since that could indeed be thyroid imbalance.

ARE YOU DIAGNOSED BUT INADEQUATELY TREATED?

- You may be one of the millions of Americans who have a diagnosed problem, now controlled to their doctors' satisfaction.

- Nevertheless, you may still have mental symptoms due entirely to thyroid imbalance. This is because some of the *physical symptoms* can be well treated, but the *mental symptoms* may require you to further refine your thyroid program in order to feel your best.

Feelings and Thyroid

Despite what many of us have been told, strong feelings can be a positive force in our lives. Though we are not often reminded of this, our feelings are actually a gift, helping us to determine whether to move toward or away from certain situations. They can warn us about danger and repel us from it. When we are in balance, our feelings can be our best guide.

- **However, when our feelings are unstable and out of our control, they can lead us to disastrous decisions and consequences.** Then, rather than guiding us, our feelings may impel us into negative behaviors, with unpleasant and sometimes dangerous results. (Davis)
- **Many people with thyroid dysfunction have, as a side effect, uncomfortable feelings that rule their lives**, distance their friendships, hurt others, and often cannot be controlled.
- **There is a surprisingly close relationship between feelings, behaviors, and thyroid function.**

Toward a New Definition of Mental Health

We want to reveal what we have learned on this journey toward better thyroid mental health care.

Troublesome feelings and behaviors are often a result of chemical reactions in the brain under the direct control of important hormones, primarily thyroid. Learning to manage our biochemical urges and to master their effects is a worthy endeavor, often with far-reaching benefit.

> **How much depression, irritability, quick anger, outright rage, and frequent panic are actually due to an easy-to-treat thyroid imbalance?**

This is not an easy question to answer. It is an issue we struggle with every day while working with hundreds of poorly treated thyroid patients. For us, as health practitioners, two things are certain:

1. People are most apt to repeat dysfunctional familial patterns *when they have not been given proper support* to transcend and replace them with healthier behaviors.

2. More relevant to this book, many people seem to have a **genetic biochemical predisposition** toward fear and anxiety, anger and rage, sadness and depression. This genetic predisposition is often mediated through autoimmunity, directed against the thyroid, resulting in gland imbalance. (Weiner)

Fortunately, this can be well treated with simple and inexpensive oral medicines.

Mind-Body-Thyroid: A Mental Health Tool

In light of the mind-body paradigm explained in Chapter 1, let us now look more carefully for the chemical causes behind human emotions. When we combine psychology with brain chemistry, we can better explore the whole person and help her to fix whatever is driving her astray.

When a person is viewed in her chemical and hormonal totality, not only can her actions be better understood, but also they may be more properly anticipated and managed. Does it take more time? Perhaps. Is it worth it? Absolutely.

Anna's Story

Anna, 43 years old, exhibited a lifelong pattern of becoming extremely anxious and agitated whenever she had to deal with her family. At an early age, she had moved far from them, trying to maintain her relationships by attending only a few selected family celebrations.

Before these events, she would become increasingly insomniac, agitated, anxious, and upset. Her husband found her very difficult at these times, and he eventually asked us if she could be helped, especially since there were two family events scheduled in the next few months.

After evaluation at our clinic, we determined that Anna had mild low thyroid causing a compensatory rise in her adrenal hormones. This resulted in an exaggerated hair-trigger response to the common stress of family reunions.

(continued)

> Once Anna started on some high-quality natural products (high doses of selenium and vitamin D for thyroid boosting, the herb valerian for relaxation, and the amino acid GABA for better sleep and relaxation), she was able to interact with family much more appropriately. It could have been predicted that without this additional hormonal balance, another family reunion would well have been ruined, certainly for Anna and her husband.

There are many other examples of useful nutritional supplements, which were first thought by doctors to be unscientific, but eventually have become part of good regular medical care. Here are a few:

- Vitamin B_6 added to the regimen of INH antibiotic for tuberculosis
- Coenzyme Q_{10} added to the regimen of statin medicines to help in the fight against high cholesterol
- High-dose folic acid (a B vitamin) added to pregnancy regimens to prevent neural tube birth deformities

Similarly, thyroid hormone function can be enhanced with well-chosen nutritional supplements. (Mason)

What We Can Learn

The psychiatric textbooks and literature are replete with descriptions of mental symptoms that appear to be partly or wholly related to thyroid hormone imbalance. In fact, there is a very rich and diverse literature on the direct relationship between thyroid disorder and a wide variety of psychiatric disorders. (Baruch)

Despite this known connection, most psychiatrists and psychologists tend to assume that the primary care doctor will have already ordered a thyroid test and therefore will have ruled out thyroid illness as the cause of mental or psychological symptoms. This, unfortunately, is not always the case.

Likewise, medical textbooks and journals offer an unusually rich and diverse literature on the direct relationship between the medical illness of "altered thyroid function" and its many psychological symptoms. Despite this, many primary providers, including general practitioners, nurse practitioners, and internists, will quickly treat a psychological symptom with a psychiatric medication, rather than perform a more complete thyroid evaluation to arrive at a more correct diagnosis.

Better thyroid care does take time, but it is worth it.

Many primary care doctors are also quick to refer the person to psychiatry, to relegate mental symptoms to be handled by a "specialist" in that area. Again, this is an unfortunate flow of events, if the result is further misdiagnosis of an underlying thyroid problem.

Regular medical doctors should know by now, since it has been part of every doctor's training, that *deficiencies in thyroid hormone produce major abnormalities* in growth, development, reproduction, and especially function of the central nervous system.

If your physician is open-minded but clearly not knowledgeable about these thyroid situations, you may wish to consider talking to your doctor about more testing and even a clinical trial of thyroid hormone. If your physician is too busy or not open to your suggestions, consider making the switch to a thyroid-friendly doctor in your area.

Autoimmune Thyroid and Brain Research: A History

Mental and psychological problems related to thyroid issues can be short-lived or sometimes long-enduring. Especially problematic are thyroid-hormone-related problems in the brain that escape detection by present methods of diagnosing thyroid levels in the rest of the body.

A major breakthrough in detection occurred in 1986, when the T3 nuclear receptor was identified. One major site of thyroid hormone action is inside the nucleus of the cell, where the DNA genetic material is read. This discovery opened up new perspectives regarding how thyroid hormone could so dramatically influence brain function.

Underscoring the importance of thyroid to brain function is research that demonstrates that the brain is more dependent on thyroid hormone than is any other organ. How important might this be in considering the large number and wide variety of mental problems?

Several good control studies have indicated that endocrine disorders in general, and thyroid imbalances in particular, are the most frequent medical conditions causing or worsening behavioral symptoms.

Hampering this line of research has been the **inability to measure thyroid hormone activity in the brain itself**. Instead, we must rely on measurement of thyroid hormone in the circulation of the body. Even the useful physical body indicators of thyroid hormone effects, such as ankle reflex or skin temperature, are only crude and indirect measures of thyroid hormone activity in the brain. Thus, the rest of the body could have normal enough thyroid levels, but the brain might be too high or too low.

Also keep in mind that most thyroid imbalance has been found to be autoimmune. The abnormal immune response itself may have important behavioral consequences. In this case the mental symptoms of thyroid illness might also occur in what doctors would consider a "normal" thyroid state. The regular blood tests and physical exam of a brain-altered thyroid sufferer might be completely normal.

Much of this research has been about the very common *hypo*thyroidism. The less common *hyper*thyroidism has even more dramatic psychological effects. The earliest example in the medical literature dates back to Caleb Parry's original report, made in 1786. He noted that fear seemed to play a role in precipitating the condition, and that people with this illness have a propensity for "morbid determinations."

A decade later the famous Irish physician Dr. Robert James Graves would describe the condition of hyperthyroidism in detail. Dr. Graves agreed completely with Parry's thinking, but added that the condition seemed also to be associated with "globus hystericus" in women. The condition he described has henceforth been called Graves' disease.

In the early 1900s, it was generally believed that cases of endocrine abnormalities were brought on by extreme stress. A research project of 1927 found a clear history of "psychic trauma as an exciting cause" in 85% of more than 3,000 cases of goiter.

Thyroid-Brain Connections

Today a variety of psychological symptoms are known to be direct effects of the excess thyroid hormone present in hyperthyroidism. These include psychotic reactions, delirium, extreme agitation, and paranoia. In many patients, these behaviors closely correlate with the circulating levels of thyroid hormone. The behavior and mental states improve when the hyperthyroid state is treated properly. Currently that involves the use of beta-blockers, thyroid-lowering nutritional remedies, and thyroid-decreasing prescription medicines to help reduce anxiety and agitation.

Psychiatrists tend to describe these symptoms as a result of a primary psychiatric disorder. Often, however, all of these symptoms will go away with proper treatment of the thyroid condition. Therefore, in these cases, such symptoms are simply an expression of a thyroid problem. Even the associated agoraphobia, social phobia, and panic attacks frequently reported in people with hyperthyroidism are not really a psychiatric panic disorder, but rather a thyroid dysfunction.

Commonly, the high thyroid state seems to coincide with a state of mania. Although it is possible that these two relatively common illnesses occur together by chance, it has been shown over and over again that the mania is basically a symptom of the hyperthyroidism.

In this same way, the frequent coexistence of thyroid imbalance and bipolar disorder might be looked at with a fresh view. Perhaps bipolar disorder is partly a "physical" illness in some people. In other words, these cases of bipolar disorder might represent psychological symptoms of a physical illness, best treated by an endocrinologist. Or is it still a severe psychological illness best treated by a psychiatrist? Or is it both?

It may make sense to consider the thyroid as both a physical and psychiatric illness, with both types of doctors needed. It might make even more sense that in many cases this distinction between physical and psychological illness is fraught with difficulty and should be abandoned.

This is especially true in the much more common situation in which mild psychiatric symptoms are present in a person with a strong family history of thyroid problems. These people may exhibit little or no physical evidence of thyroid imbalance. What they actually may have are **psychological symptoms caused by their medical problem**. Recall that the research shows thyroid-caused psychiatric symptoms can often be present in the absence of obvious thyroid abnormality. (Hatotani)

Recall, too, that depression, impaired concentration, and irritability are the thyroid's most common mental symptoms. Also seen, however, are mania and psychotic thought. These severe symptoms are less common, but just as frequently misdiagnosed. These can all occur as a direct result of thyroid abnormality, especially in people whose psychotherapy or psychiatric medication is not very successful. In a great many of these cases, treatment with thyroid hormone proves very helpful.

These people, with only mental symptoms of undiagnosed thyroid imbalance, pose several questions. What shall we ultimately call their condition? How common might it be? Health care consumers would feel more comfortable if the situation were more clear-cut. If tests indeed showed hypothyroidism, with few physical symptoms but definite psychological symptoms, then most practitioners would call it hypothyroidism with prominent mental symptoms.

Now imagine the same scenario, but with normal thyroid tests. (Remember that people can have a troublesome autoimmune thyroid even with normal thyroid blood tests.) What would you call it and what would you do when the tests are normal for these people?

Levels of thyroid hormone that can be measured in the circulation (blood testing) offer only a statistical relationship to metabolic activity. Any given target tissues, such as the brain, may be functionally either hypo- or hyperthyroid, in the context of these normal test results. (Joffe)

There is actually a diagnosis called "subclinical hypothyroidism," which means the patient appears to have no symptoms of thyroid problems at all, except that on blood testing there are higher-than-normal levels of TSH, a pituitary hormone, suggesting a need for more thyroid hormone. A number of research projects have linked subclinical hypothyroidism with depression.

- Subclinical hypothyroidism is believed to exist in perhaps 10% of the population, with greater than 20% for women over age 60. In this population, it is common to find what psychiatrists call "refractory depression," a type of depression not well ameliorated or successfully treated by standard depression pharmacology. (Gewirtz)

- **Another researcher found almost 20% to 33% of subclinical thyroid problems in depressed women.** This means that about 20% to 33% of female depression might be thyroid caused, representing a lot of women who have been put on Prozac instead of getting the thyroid they need.

- It was way back in 1873 when a physician commented on the mental status of a hypothyroid patient. Sir William Gull described the **hypothyroid patient as having a slowness of thought and a**

lessening of nervous power, with changes in temper and tendency for "lacissitude," or lack of motivation.

- More than 10 years later, a classic report on low thyroid from the
Clinical Society of London pointed out that **16 of 45 severely low
thyroid patients carried a diagnosis of insanity, most exhibiting
delusions and hallucinations.** This report of 1888, nicknamed
"Myxedema Madness," included descriptions of a very large range
of psychiatric and personality disturbances.

- Other reports soon followed. In one group of patients with **rapid-
cycling bipolar disorder, more than 50% were classified as having hypothyroidism.** Since then to the present day, it has been clear
that thyroid illness frequently presents with psychiatric symptoms.
It is common to see presentations in which change in mood and
mental faculty totally accompany change in thyroid function.

- **Retardation, delusions, mood disorder, and delirium should be
added to the long list of thyroid-caused mental symptoms.** Overall, according to most researchers who have studied this carefully,
the thyroid represents the best naturally occurring model for inves-
tigating the biochemical mechanisms for mood and brain function.

Thyroid's Central Role
in Mental Health

Good internists know from published reports, as well as their clinical
practices, that most patients with severe hypothyroidism also suffer from
depression.

How many people with depression suffer from it because of hypothyroidism? Some researchers feel this could be as high as 50%. Others suggest
40% or 30%—still a significant portion.

Depression is only one of the many thyroid-related psychiatric illnesses. Many researchers suggest others, including attention deficit disorder (ADD), attention-deficit/hyperactivity disorder (ADHD), seasonal
affective disorder (SAD), alcoholism, eating disorders, autism, and even low
libido and erectile dysfunction. (Nemeroff)

This list is so extensive that many neuroscientists have come to view
the thyroid gland as an "annex to the brain," since the brain uses thyroid

chemicals for such a wide variety of normal brain functions. Overall, therefore, thyroid hormone balance in the brain is crucial for maintaining stable mood, emotions, and behavior.

Depression and anxiety disorders are the most common psychiatric conditions in the general population; they also happen to be the *most common mental effects of thyroid disease.* Many of the symptoms of these heretofore understood as psychological maladies can be controlled through correcting thyroid brain chemistry. Thyroid hormone can help depressed and anxious patients stabilize their brain chemistry when conventional antidepressant therapy has failed. (Arem)

A recent article explored cases of hypothyroidism presenting as psychosis: "Hypothyroidism is a potential cause for multiple psychological disturbances . . . The realization that thyroid abnormalities might be the potential cause of an assortment of symptoms is critical in the proper identification and treatment of the patients." (Heinrich)

What You Can Do

Thyroid malfunction needs to be considered more often, and more carefully, as the possible cause of psychological illness. This is not a new view, but it is one that needs further recognition and attention by practicing physicians, alternative practitioners, and especially the lay public.

> We encourage you—as empowered health consumers—to be attuned to the likelihood that the thyroid could be a factor in *any* mental health concerns.

Talk to your health practitioner about checking this connection very thoroughly. If you have a practitioner who does not seem to care that you may have an underlying thyroid disorder causing psychological distress, you may want to find someone different to work with on this specific aspect of your health journey.

Another option to consider is the exciting newly available resource where you can self-order your own complete, highly accurate panel of thyroid tests: www.CanaryClub.org. More thorough recommendations for how to do this are given in the next chapter.

> You may be asking why most doctors haven't been testing more carefully for this rampant thyroid epidemic.

As a health consumer, it's incumbent upon you to enlighten your practitioners so that you get better thyroid care. You can insist on more accurate thyroid testing, with more open-minded interpretation, if not with your present practitioner, then with one willing to listen, learn, and help you better. At times it seems that health consumers in our present system are not encouraged to become more aware of the many connections that help us to understand and improve our lives. Yet the very quality, and sometimes quantity, of our lives is dependent upon this very skill: our ability to listen, to synthesize information, to trust our own instincts, and to speak out.

Jeff's Story

Jeff is a local presence in our town, a storyteller and teacher who has traveled and practiced yoga, meditation, mind control, and other Eastern religion pursuits. He'd always been in excellent control of his thoughts and emotions.

At age 58, however, for no apparent reason, he was gripped by a gradual and unexpected onset of negativity, discomfort, and doubt. His internal sense of himself as a well-balanced person was suddenly slipping away, replaced by a more anxious and disorganized self.

A less knowledgeable person might have felt that he was losing his mind. His thoughts and feelings were coming rapid fire. His focus would jump from one aspect of his life to another, seemingly at random. This was a totally new experience for him.

Jeff's observation of his own mental process was that it was now like a swarm of bees flying around, finally alighting in one crook of a tree. His thoughts would briefly settle on one particular aspect of his life, such as an upcoming job change, finances, health concerns, or the car needing gas. Then, just as quickly, he would start thinking about something entirely different and unrelated. This seemed bizarre even as he watched himself.

Rather than obsess or worry about this new phenomenon that was asserting itself into a previously disciplined mind, he realized there must be something wrong. Despite a complete lack of physical symptoms, he went to a doctor of internal medicine, not a mental specialist, asking what physical problem might be causing these psychological symptoms.

(continued)

Many tests came back normal, but one was mildly out of balance—his thyroid level. It was just barely in the hyperthyroid range. With proper treatment of his high thyroid situation, the mental experience of losing his mind went completely away.

This is a good example of proactive self-care. Others may have spent an uncomfortably long time being treated with psychological medicine or psychotherapy, to little or no avail.

A high index of suspicion for thyroid problems is quite useful in these varied situations.

Jeff is doing quite well now. He expressed a strong desire to let others know just how forceful and compelling these feelings were. They were gripping, taking over his life to the exclusion of all else. He now has great sympathy for people going through thyroid problems, especially those who have yet to uncover the true reason for their psychological and mental symptoms.

Please know that we do *not* believe that most people have thyroid disease, *nor* that most people showing mental symptoms have the thyroid as the cause.

We are simply making you aware of a few simple yet neglected facts:

- A significant percentage of the population could receive better care more quickly, and at much lower cost, for many life-threatening conditions, *if only they were properly evaluated* for having even a mild thyroid condition.

- Many *could be spared more debilitating symptoms* down the road if this type of low-level, energy-draining condition were addressed earlier, rather than being allowed to smolder and grow.

- *Fixing it early is easy*; fixing it later is much more difficult, when its damage is not fully reversible and after it has been causing havoc in your systems for years.

- Because the simpler T4 and TSH blood determinations are notoriously inaccurate, you could have the brain effects of thyroid imbalance, even with normal test results.

Complementary Healing for Your Best Results

By Georjana Shames, LAc

Deficiencies in thyroid hormone can produce major abnormalities in development, reproduction, growth, and especially function of the central nervous system. In classical Acupuncture theory, Chinese physicians did not use the words *thyroid deficiency*, but rather would describe a corresponding aspect of the human system, such as "Kidney Meridian Xu" (deficiency of the Kidney Meridian).

The Kidney Meridian is the root of the body's energy, closely corresponding to what in Western medicine is considered thyroid and adrenal function.

- When hypothyroidism is diagnosed in Western medicine, it most often (but not always) corresponds to a diagnosis of deficiency of Kidney Yang in Acupuncture theory. Hypothyroid patients often feel sluggish and exhausted, which makes sense, as they lack Kidney Yang, the warming, invigorating energy.

- When hyperthyroidism is diagnosed in Western medicine, it most often (but not always) corresponds to a deficiency of Kidney Yin. Hyperthyroid patients often feel overwrought and full of nervous anxiety, which makes sense, as they lack Kidney Yin, the calming, cooling energy.

In Chinese Medicine, the brain corresponds to what we call the Sea of Marrow, which encompasses the spinal cord and the brain itself. The Sea of Marrow can be thought of as a metaphor and representation of robust mental acuity. When all is not well, you can imagine that the sea is at low tide, and mental function decreases.

Abundant Kidney Meridian energy nourishes and builds the Sea of Marrow. We know for a fact that a deficiency in the Kidney Meridian will result in failure to nourish the Sea of Marrow, so we can draw a direct link in Acupuncture theory between thyroid hormone deficiency and mental symptoms in the patient.

The patient can be depressed, anxious, foggy-headed, not thinking clearly, and having trouble with deduction and with appropriate behaviors.

In Acupuncture the Shen, or the Spirit, is integral to our ability to behave appropriately in any given situation. Therefore, we can see that the **more extreme versions of mental illness** (bipolar, paranoia, etc.) can be **closely linked to a disturbance of the Mind and the Spirit**.

On a less extreme level, we find that a person with inability to utilize the Kidney Meridian's energy (which we call Qi) or essence (which we call Jing) can show a mild form of depression or emotional detachment, causing them to behave in ways that are not fully relating to the outer world and to situations around them.

The common example of a woman who has given birth and now has postpartum depression, stemming from a previous thyroid deficiency that had gone undiagnosed and untreated for many years, relates in Acupuncture theory to the lack of nourishment from the Kidney Meridian deficiency. The new mother has given her Blood, Jing, and Qi to the cause of gestation and birth of this infant. She does not have enough left over after the baby's birth to nourish herself internally; thus she becomes despondent, the Sea of Marrow is not nourished, her mental acuity decreases, and her behavior changes. She can become severely unhappy and irrationally angry at the infant, and she may even reject her child.

This is an extreme example of a common problem: **if you do not nourish yourself, you will have nothing left to give to the others in your life**. If there is nothing internally to sustain you, you are unable to give to another human being what you also lack.

In general, lack of energy coursing through the Kidney Meridian could be caused by a congenital deficiency, a life of stress, a difficult trauma that was never resolved, very poor nutrition, a sedentary lifestyle, and so on. We find then that a person is unable to produce internally the qualities and substances required for proper nourishment of the brain and glands. He or she may become exhausted, overwhelmed with emotional and mental symptoms of anxiety, depression, and lapses in memory.

One reason that a person might be able to have a low thyroid condition that manifests only in mental or emotional symptoms is that the body is very good at compensating, perhaps better than the mind is. The physical drive to live and reproduce is integral to every aspect of our survival as a species. So it is quite possible that mental symptoms are more prominent or more prevalent earlier. **Before the body becomes exhausted, the mind can become exhausted.**

The Sea of Marrow is not being nourished by the Kidney Meridian's Blood, Jing, and Qi, and the body can continue overworking under too much stress temporarily, allowing the adrenals to compensate for a low thyroid condition temporarily. The person's mental health suffers, as energy is being diverted away from the mind and into propelling the physical ability to survive.

Over time, a deficiency of the Kidney Meridian (relating to the body's energy) or a deficiency of the Spleen Meridian (relating to extracting fuel from your food during digestion) ultimately can fail to produce enough nourishment for the Heart Meridian, which in Acupuncture theory houses the Mind.

In a domino effect, one deficiency eventually creates another deficiency.

The Sea of Marrow (the brain) and the Heart Meridian (housing the Mind) are not being nourished by the Kidney energy, leaving a deficit. Those deficits lead to:

- A lack of mental clarity
- An inability to speak one's mind in an articulate way
- Difficulty with overwhelming emotions

This shows you how, in Acupuncture theory, a thyroid imbalance can actually cause or exacerbate a mental imbalance.

THE BOTTOM LINE

- Thyroid imbalance is just one brain factor that strongly affects mind and emotions. There are many other known physical causes of psychological illness.
- Chemical toxicity, brain tumors, and degenerative nervous system diseases are examples of nonthyroid-caused mental imbalance. We hope the public becomes more aware of the importance of identifying these other known causes and evaluating them properly.
- In addition to these known causes, there are many unknown reasons for aberrant behavior. The great master Freud himself started off his medical career as a physical doctor, a neurologist. Even in his later life as a mental specialist, Freud told his students repeatedly that eventually the physical causes of most mental conditions would be found. These physical conditions could be treated much more efficaciously than relying strictly on psychiatric interventions.

Well, Dr. Freud, we are happy to tell you that here is one of the larger physical causes of mental illness: thyroid.

This thyroid issue is compelling and worthy of much closer attention, especially in our country's ongoing health care debate. This is not only because thyroid problems are so increasingly common in our polluted world but also because they are so easy and inexpensive to treat. Treating thyroid first can save you years of chasing mental symptoms.

RECOMMENDED ACTION PLAN

- Realize that thyroid issues can be the root cause of *any* long-standing psychological issues.

- Know that **optimal treatment of thyroid imbalance** can provide additional **relief** from depression, anxiety, loss of memory and focus, sleep problems, or harmful habits.

3

Is Thyroid Causing YOUR Symptoms?

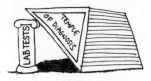

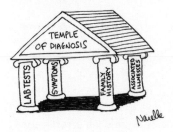

Narelle

Lucy's Story

Lucy Johnson was at the breaking point. A single mom with two toddlers, she always had too much to do. Today, somehow, it was worse, much worse. Because her babysitter had not shown up, she was forced to tell the office she was sick and would miss a crucial meeting.

She no longer cared about the meeting, or anything else for that matter; it was all just too much. She collapsed on the couch, oblivious to

(continued)

her kids—or where they were playing. They had slowly migrated from the living room, out the front door, across the yard, somehow unlatched the gate, and were ambling closer and closer to the steep-sided canal.

How had her life become so precarious? For this past year she had known something was very wrong. She had gone to her HMO repeatedly, only to be told that they could see nothing abnormal in her exam or lab tests. Even an expensive private doctor had found nothing. They all reassured her that busy working moms are often tired. Meanwhile, Lucy kept getting seriously more fatigued and fuzzy-headed.

She had briefly wondered why, today, it had suddenly gotten to the point where she felt like an electric lamp whose plug had been pulled. Part of her knew that she could no longer hear the kids playing in the yard, but she was unable to get up or call out for them.

The children had decided that Mommy's nap was their chance to go swimming. When a passerby heard screaming, he ran to the canal and pulled out one child, who was visible. Police later retrieved the body of the second.

The tragedy that changed this family forever was senseless and unnecessary. It later was determined that Lucy had been in a near-comatose condition from severe hypothyroidism. The TSH level, the only blood test all her doctors had used to check for thyroid imbalance, was not sufficient for the task. It had shown normal, but Lucy's metabolism had not been normal at all.

The bigger tragedy is that this type of thyroid lab error is not at all unusual. Careful researchers estimate that millions of people are experiencing a degraded quality of life from an undue faith in the overrated TSH test. Most of the time this can amount to years of annoyance. Sometimes, however, it is the difference between life and death.

Standard Testing Concerns

Suppose you suspect that a thyroid abnormality is at the root of some of your mental symptoms. How would you go about proving this to the satisfaction of a practitioner, who could write you a prescription for the condition and work alongside you to determine your progress?

The standard answer to this question is to have your general practice physician, internist, nurse practitioner, or gynecologist order a TSH test. There actually are several different thyroid tests, but TSH is now considered the "gold standard," unfortunately for many thyroid sufferers.

TSH, or thyroid-stimulating hormone testing, has gained enough favor on the part of enough doctors in recent years that it is now considered the *one standard procedure* to rule in, or rule out, thyroid problems. You simply go to a blood lab, stick out your arm, have the TSH test drawn, and then wait for the result.

If the result shows a thyroid abnormality, then you have a thyroid problem. If the result doesn't show a thyroid abnormality, then you've ruled it out. Right?

There is one serious problem with all of this.

This standard test, TSH, while very useful for severe thyroid problems, is *woefully inadequate* for diagnosing most thyroid conditions.

TSH can be helpful for identifying easy-to-diagnose thyroid problems, but it is **not a useful maneuver for most people**, especially for those who seek to determine if thyroid is the cause of their mental symptoms.

Why is this TSH test inadequate?

The one TSH test is simply *not sensitive enough* to diagnose the milder forms of thyroid dysfunction, which is what most people have.

More people have milder forms of thyroid imbalance. While not as dramatic, milder imbalances can still contribute to many types of psychological disturbance.

Tragically, most doctors only look for serious thyroid problems. People who are suffering from less obvious thyroid conditions are essentially told to go home and live their lives. These people are often who we see in our clinic, after years of chasing symptoms, being denied, and feeling drained.

If you have symptoms or strong family history of thyroid, and you wish to reclaim your life, do not allow a TSH test alone to be used as your complete thyroid evaluation.

Even though the name of the test is the "sensitive TSH test" or "highly sensitive TSH test," even if called "the newer ultra-sensitive TSH test," don't let the name fool you.

The tests are not as sensitive as they need to be.

This test is not, on its own, a wholly reliable indicator of your thyroid status.

A Better Way to Check Your Thyroid

We recommend adding a panel of thyroid tests. Below we have included our preferred testing panel.

The panel of tests should include a measurement of the following:

- TSH
- Free T4
- Free T3
- Two thyroid antibody tests:
  - Thyroid peroxidase antibody (TPO)
  - Thyroglobulin antibody (TG antibody)

With additional tests added to the TSH, you now have a much more complete picture of what is actually going on with various aspects of your thyroid function.

Today you can self-order, knowing perhaps better than your doctor does that you need help. The Canary Club (www.CanaryClub.org) has a variety of self-testing maneuvers that can help to make sure you get all the tests you need *for a more accurate diagnosis*.

Simply join, free of charge. You can then self-order in the lab testing section (ZRT central lab's AdvancedPlus Panel). Your kit will arrive with complete instructions for testing your sex hormones and adrenal hormones.

- You start by capturing your early morning, late morning, mid-afternoon, and bedtime saliva samples, which are then tested for cortisol levels, as well as sex hormones (estriol, estradiol, progesterone, and testosterone). (While at the time of publication thyroid testing by saliva is still considered "experimental," we have found this method to be of great value.)
- In addition, the kit includes a spring-loaded sterile lance used to puncture your finger and help you obtain blood from the periphery, which we feel is **more accurate than blood taken from the vein.**

To start with Canary Club, we suggest you obtain the AdvancedPlus Panel. This gives a quick onetime baseline test for 12 related hormones (from thyroid, adrenal, and sex glands) as well as for vitamin D. It costs around $225 as of the timing of this project and has helped thousands like you to get exactly the answers they were seeking.

If you would like to self-order but would prefer to use blood testing, there are new options for this as well. See "Our Testing Recommendations" in the Appendix at the back of the book for the most current information on how you can order your own tests to check for hormones.

Hints for Better Interpretation of Your Tests

In addition to getting sufficient testing, there is also the controversial issue of test interpretation. Here are some aspects to consider first.

Range of Normal Issues

Consider the TSH test as a prime example: since the early 2000s, the American Association of Clinical Endocrinologists (AACE, the main endocrine specialists society in the United States) has been suggesting to its members and other interested practitioners that a new range of normal is necessary for proper evaluation of the TSH test.

The old range was 0.5 to 5.5 for many years. Until recently, people who fell between the 3.0 and 5.5 range were considered normal.

Since 2002, the AACE has recommended that the range of normal be 0.3 to 3.0. Any TSH above 3.0 is highly suspicious for thyroid abnormality.

In other words, to all those millions who have been told by their doctors for years, "Your thyroid is normal," here's what you got:

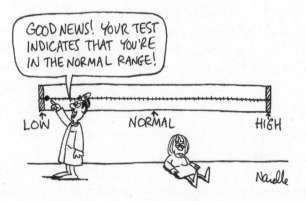

This scenario has continued for far too long. The only missing ingredient has been *you*—the Empowered Health Consumer. We cannot just blame doctors; most are so overwrought and undernourished that they do what is quick, easy, and acceptable. Surely nurses cannot be at fault. Since the inception, nurses have been trying to support physicians yet empower consumers to improve health delivery.

Now, it is up to consumers to help create a new era, one in which the patient is the main decision maker, guided by other health professionals, both allopathic and integrative . . . for one simple reason: **it's your life!**

Blood Examination Options

Keep in mind that the **type of blood** being used for the test can strongly influence the result.

Venous blood, the standard blood drawn from the crook of the arm, is not as accurate as capillary blood, drawn from a fingertip, for hormonal evaluation. There are several reasons for this, related to the capillary blood remaining more stable in terms of the information being delivered to cells and tissues.

Capillary blood from a quick finger stick is immediately dried on a piece of special filter paper, fixing the specimen so the amount of TSH is stable until the test is actually run.

The blood drawn from a vein in the arm is kept as *liquid serum*, usually all day. This blood, probably drawn in the morning, is then driven by a courier to a central location where, later on, it is run through large automated machinery, often at night.

During this time, the TSH—a fragile pituitary hormone—will have degraded; less of it will be available in the tube to be detected on determination equipment. **The result, therefore, is not as accurate**, because some of the material you were trying to measure as a liquid in the test tube has degraded while waiting to be run.

Other reasons that capillary blood is a better test are that it is much more convenient, less painful, less time consuming, and less expensive.

We Need Better Tests

Even when doing the best blood tests, using the best ranges of normal to interpret the results, we still find the current state of the art is lacking.

No amount of blood testing is necessarily sufficient for proper determination of the presence of a thyroid abnormality. In other words:

You could still be low or high thyroid, *even with normal blood tests.*

We do not yet have tests to show how much thyroid hormone is available to the brain, or how efficiently thyroid hormone is being utilized in the brain. This is really what you want to know. To date, all thyroid testing, as presently performed, only answers that question indirectly.

In addition to these challenges in testing, there are other issues that must be addressed. One is resistance to thyroid hormone. There are also thyroid antibodies that may or may not be detected, which could affect how well the hormone is doing its job in the brain tissue.

It is *not* enough to perform blood tests, find that results are normal, then say, "That rules out any chance of a thyroid problem." It doesn't.

The bottom line is that you could still have a thyroid problem, even with normal tests. Unless the blood tests positively show the issue—you can trust that, since thyroid tests have very few false positives—other diagnostic maneuvers, in addition to blood testing, need to be included.

If the test shows positive, you can rely on it. If the test shows normal or negative, you may rightfully question it, or explore further.

Additional Diagnostic Methods

Along with blood or saliva testing, include a careful and complete:

- Evaluation of your psychological and physical symptoms
- Evaluation of who in your *family had thyroid* problems or *autoimmune issues* related to thyroid (diabetes or rheumatoid arthritis)
- Evaluation of your related conditions and evaluation of your physical signs

Family History

If your family has other autoimmune issues, you could have a thyroid problem, regardless of what blood tests show.

Thyroid is one of the most, if not *the* most inherited of all medical conditions.

If anybody in your family, especially a close relative, has had *any* thyroid issue, then you could be genetically inclined toward a thyroid issue.

This can mean it would be helpful for you to check whether Aunt Tillie or Uncle Joe ever had a thyroid problem, either now or in the past.

- Whether or not your mother's struggles with fatigue, depression, or weight may have been thyroid related is important for you to know.
- If her tests ever showed abnormal or even borderline, or if there were ever any thyroid nodules, you need to know this.
- If there ever was enlargement of the gland, called a *goiter*, knowing this could be very useful to you as well.
- These taken together may all point to a diagnosis more definitive than would normal blood tests alone.

Keep in mind that for many people in your family, a thyroid issue may not be considered a medical problem. Here is an example of an exchange that seems typical of our patients over the years:

"Did you ever have any medical problems, Grandma?"

"No," says Grandma.

"Grandma, did you ever take any medicine for a medical problem?"

"No," says Grandma.

And then you point out a bottle of thyroid pills in the medicine chest and say, "Grandma, what's this?"

"Oh, that," says Grandma. "That's just my thyroid. That's nothing. I've been taking one of those a day for years. That's not a medical problem, that's just my thyroid."

Many of their relatives do not consider thyroid, and thyroid medicine, an actual medical issue. It is such a minor aspect of their lives that they often do not even consider writing it down on a medical form when asked their health history.

For all of these reasons, thyroid has been called the great masquerader. With the help of *Thyroid Mind Power*, you will be able to uncover it.

At the end of this chapter, we will present questions about your family history, as well as your own medical history. If you had a thyroid problem as a teenager but have "grown out of it," that may point to the possibility that you have a thyroid issue now. It may be mild and under the surface, yet still causing psychological symptoms.

Related Conditions

There are a number of medical situations whose presence increases the likelihood that you have a thyroid issue. Something as simple as having carpal tunnel syndrome, having gray hair early in life, or even being left-handed can each be significant in pointing the way to an otherwise elusive diagnosis. The questionnaire at the end of this chapter will ask about these "related conditions."

Physical Signs

When we speak of "physical signs," we are talking about detectable aspects that are not necessarily symptoms, yet could cause a person to complain.

A typical physical sign is your body temperature. You may not feel particularly hot or particularly cold, but if you take your temperature with a good basal thermometer, you might find that you are above or below normal.

Thyroid controls temperature.

A list of physical signs appears in the questionnaire at the end of this chapter. We suggest you consider these signs carefully and answer the questions honestly.

Once your attention is called to a physical sign, you might become more aware of it. Paying attention earlier can avert future problems.

Refining the Art of Temperature Taking

Since the physical sign of temperature is one of the most important and commonly measured, it deserves some special attention here prior to the questionnaire.

A good reason to measure your temperature is to see if your basal metabolic rate is adequate, too low, or too high.

The best time to measure is in the morning, right after you wake up, before you get out of bed. You are awake, but you don't stir. Best to have shaken your thermometer down low the evening before, so you do not have to move even that much. Taking your temperature upon waking approximates the sleeping temperature, which is one measure of your basal metabolic rate. Remember that metabolism is how we ingest, digest, and expel our foods to release energy into our system.

Always take your temperature with a very accurate **basal thermometer**, preferably nonmercury filled (see Resources). An accurate measurement can be found using the armpit, which is easy to access. Leave the thermometer in for at least 5 minutes to fully equilibrate.

An electronic thermometer does not take this long before signaling to you that it is ready for you to read the temperature. We mention the 5 minutes of time because we recommend a nondigital basal thermometer. Newer ones use a nonmercury liquid. If they are indeed marked "basal," they are generally more accurate than the more expensive electronic variety.

For people who have any inflammation of the oral cavity, ears, nose, or sinuses, it might be best to put the thermometer somewhere other than the mouth. A rectal reading is highly accurate, but most people would prefer putting the thermometer bulb in the armpit, arm comfortably at the side.

Again, keep the **thermometer there for at least 5 minutes** to allow for equilibration, and then make your readings. The comparisons in the questionnaires at the end of this chapter will help you decide whether you are in the normal range or too high or too low (< 97.6 average = low).

Questionnaires

It is soon time to answer your four-part questionnaire, considering:

- Your psychological and physical symptoms
- Your family history
- Your related conditions
- Your physical signs

The purpose of this questionnaire is to create a more complete evaluation than can be made by blood testing alone.

If blood tests show that you *do have a thyroid problem*, you do not need to complete these other steps using questionnaires, although you might find these evaluations quite interesting.

If, on the other hand, your *blood tests are normal*, but you do not feel like your old self, you would definitely want to evaluate these four areas more carefully. The lack of diagnosis, and the resulting lack of treatment, can result in continued needless suffering.

Your current mental symptoms might indeed still be thyroid related. They may well be thyroid related, even with normal tests. If you measure your score against the scoring key at the very end of the chapter, you will have a chance to make a "presumptive diagnosis," regardless of blood tests.

Then what?

Once you have made a presumptive diagnosis, you might want to consider a trial of over-the-counter thyroid remedies. Depending on how well these work, you may next want to do a trial of prescription thyroid medicine.

Chapters 4 through 8 describe specific kinds of mental issues caused by thyroid abnormality, and also detail what kinds of remedies and medicines we most recommend. Many people who suffer from thyroid conditions correspond to particular "types" such as moody, edgy, foggy, sleepy, and needy.

Chapters 9 and 10 explore types of over-the-counter remedies that do not require a doctor's prescription. They also address those products available only through prescription by licensed practitioners.

We wish you very good luck in arriving at a proper diagnosis.

Remember, thyroid tests do not replace good clinical judgment, and should not be used alone to confirm or refute a diagnostic impression, or to dictate therapy.

Here we can also share some particular hints that might be useful. Suppose you have a depression being treated with antidepressants, but you've received no benefit from the antidepressants, even after trying several. Instead, you've only experienced side effects from the antidepressants. This is a further indication that you might actually have a depression caused by thyroid abnormality.

Here's another hint: it might help if you could identify the actual time of onset of your symptoms. Whether considering your sleep problem, depression, anxiety, or memory loss, if this issue mainly started around the time of a certain event (for example, puberty, childbirth, menopause, or after an accident, illness, or surgery), you might well want to consider that the thyroid is what went off course.

The telltale sign of this is when a person says, "I haven't felt right since my knee surgery." Or, "I haven't felt like myself since that freeway fender bender." Or, "I haven't seen my usual sharp mind since that bronchitis last winter." If you have found yourself talking like this, then you may really want to think about a thyroid diagnosis quite carefully.

Also of particular importance is if any of the physical thyroid signs began around the same time as some of these mental symptoms. That could be very compelling, revealing the possibility of thyroid being an issue in your psychological makeup.

Thyroid could be the total cause of your mental symptoms, even with completely normal thyroid blood tests.

Self-Assessment Questionnaires

Here are listings of symptoms and related conditions, family history questions, and a group of physical signs. These can be of help to you in determining whether thyroid is a factor in your mental life.

To start, **check each of these that you have experienced**, then review the scoring card at the end of the questionnaires.

Symptoms of Low Thyroid

Do you have:

- ☐ Bothersome **fatigue** or weakness
- ☐ Any chronically recurring **infection**
- ☐ Regular low moods
- ☐ **Hoarseness** for no particular reason
- ☐ Difficulty swallowing
- ☐ **Decreased sweating**, even with heavy exercise
- ☐ Slowness in heating up, even in a sauna
- ☐ **Red face** with exercise
- ☐ **Constipation**, regardless of fiber and liquids
- ☐ **Nails** that crack or peel easily
- ☐ Troublesome **headaches**

- ☐ **Energy dropouts** later in the day
- ☐ Irregular menstrual periods
- ☐ Unusually low sex drive
- ☐ Mood swings
- ☐ **Gums** that are receding or that bleed easily
- ☐ Continued **weight gain**, despite good diet and exercise
- ☐ **Aches and pains** unrelated to exertion
- ☐ Severely dry skin or adult acne
- ☐ Ovarian cysts, endometriosis, miscarriage, or infertility
- ☐ Trouble with **focus**, concentration, or memory
- ☐ Excessive **hair loss**
- ☐ The sensation of feeling **colder** than other people
- ☐ Intolerance to heat
- ☐ Increasing difficulty with balance
- ☐ **Tingling** or burning sensations that come and go

Symptoms of High Thyroid

Do you have:

- ☐ People telling you that you are **staring** at them too intently
- ☐ Light or **skipped periods** (unrelated to vigorous exercise, pregnancy, or menopause)
- ☐ The sensation of feeling often like you have had too much coffee
- ☐ Fast bowels or **loose stools**
- ☐ Unexpected **weight loss** (when not on a diet)
- ☐ Experience of feeling **unusually hot** much of the time
- ☐ Breathlessness or **panic attacks** for no reason
- ☐ Excessive **anxiety**, out of place for life events
- ☐ **Extra energy**, hardly needing sleep
- ☐ Excessively **rapid heart rate** at rest
- ☐ New experience of shaking or tremor
- ☐ Skipped heartbeats or **palpitations**
- ☐ Sense of **revved-up** metabolism

- [ ] Continually warm, **moist skin**
- [ ] Unusual **irritability**, without clear cause
- [ ] Pronounced **nervousness** for no special reason

Related Conditions

Do you have:

- [ ] Prematurely **gray** hair
- [ ] Dyslexia
- [ ] Rheumatoid **arthritis**
- [ ] **Anemia** or B_{12} deficiency
- [ ] Lupus
- [ ] **Crohn's** disease
- [ ] Unusual and ongoing **visual changes**
- [ ] Sarcoidosis
- [ ] Ulcerative **colitis**
- [ ] Manic-depressive disorder (**bipolar**)
- [ ] Low blood platelets
- [ ] Scleroderma
- [ ] Mitral valve prolapse
- [ ] White or blue **discoloration of fingers** when cold (Raynaud's)
- [ ] Carpal tunnel syndrome
- [ ] Atrial fibrillation
- [ ] Sjögren's syndrome (dry eyes)
- [ ] **Losing head hair** in patches (alopecia)
- [ ] Biliary cirrhosis
- [ ] Calcium deficiency
- [ ] Attention deficit disorder (ADD)
- [ ] Endometriosis
- [ ] Neck injury such as **whiplash**
- [ ] Large white depigmented patches on the skin (**vitiligo**)
- [ ] Multiple sclerosis (MS)
- [ ] Left-handedness

Family History

Have your blood relatives ever had:

- ☐ High thyroid (**Graves'** hyperthyroid)
- ☐ Low thyroid (**Hashimoto's** hypothyroidism)
- ☐ Enlarged thyroid (**goiter**)
- ☐ Thyroid **nodules**
- ☐ Prematurely **gray** hair
- ☐ Rheumatoid **arthritis**
- ☐ Anemia or B_{12} deficiency
- ☐ Lupus
- ☐ **Crohn's** disease
- ☐ Sarcoidosis
- ☐ Ulcerative **colitis**
- ☐ Manic-depressive disorder (**bipolar**)
- ☐ Low blood platelets
- ☐ Scleroderma
- ☐ White or blue **discoloration of fingers** when cold (Raynaud's)
- ☐ **Sjögren's** syndrome (dry eyes)
- ☐ **Losing head hair** in patches (alopecia)
- ☐ Biliary cirrhosis (liver damage)
- ☐ Large white depigmented patches on the skin (**vitiligo**)
- ☐ Multiple sclerosis (MS)
- ☐ **Left-handedness**

Physical Signs

Have you or your practitioner observed:

- ☐ Noticeable **weakness**
- ☐ Recurrent **swelling** of the feet
- ☐ **Low morning basal temperature** (3-day average less than 97.6°)
- ☐ Excessive **bags under eyes** or swelling of eyelids
- ☐ **Tongue slightly swollen**; repeatedly biting it, as if too big for mouth

☐ **Slow speech,** slow movements and reaction time

☐ Pale lips, pale skin

☐ **Enlargement of the thyroid** area at the base of the neck

☐ Irregularity or asymmetry of the thyroid gland

☐ Decreased thickness of outer eyebrows

☐ **Very slow pulse,** without being in good physical shape

☐ Excessive amounts of **ear wax**

☐ Dry skin, dry mouth, dry eyes

☐ Skin that is **cool or cold** to the touch

☐ Low blood pressure

☐ Abnormally brisk or **sluggish reflexes**

Interpretation of Your Score

(Each checked box counts as 1.)

	0 to 3	Unlikely to be a thyroid issue
	4 to 7	Somewhat suspicious for thyroid issue
	8 to 11	Very suspicious for thyroid issue
	12 to 15	Likely to be a thyroid issue
	16 or more	We'll eat our hat if it's not thyroid!

Jump Start for All Mind-Types

There are many ways to begin to jump-start your thyroid function to improve your mood, memory, or sleep. One of the best places to start fixing any sluggish metabolism is to provide more of the required nutrients that fuel this process. Here are the four most important categories:

1. **Vitamins and minerals** are *co-factors acting as catalysts* in the *extraction of metabolic energy from food.* Take a *high-quality multivitamin daily,* such as Multigenics by the Metagenics company. (Take 4 each morning.)

2. The **antioxidants** *protect the body* from the wear and tear of daily living, called *oxidative stress.* Protect your thyroid

metabolism with an extra-strong antioxidant like Oxygenics, also by Metagenics (Take 1 each morning.)

3. The **omega oils** are involved in helping to *maintain the integrity of the cell membranes* and the *viability of the hormone receptors.* An excellent mix of omega-3 with omega-6 fatty acids is Omega EFA by Metagenics. (Take 1 daily.)

4. Lastly, **amino acids** are crucial in completing your jump start, since *thyroid hormone is built up from a basic amino acid structure.* Exceptional aminos can be obtained from Metagenics as BioPure Protein. Take 10 grams (1 scoop) daily of this purified protein powder.

Also keep in mind that Dr. Rich Shames can work with you by phone to help you get started on your program (www.ThyroidMindPower.com).

Complementary Healing for Your Best Results

By Georjana Shames, LAc

Acupuncture theory can help you diagnose a potential thyroid problem, especially if your lab tests are inconclusive. For many thyroid sufferers, low thyroid conditions are recognized by lab tests, and the patient is put on medication.

But, as you have gathered thus far in this book, there are a large number of people who receive "false negatives" on their thyroid tests. In other words, they **do have a thyroid condition**, but **the standard lab tests are not sensitive enough** or thorough enough to register it.

Lab tests are wonderful and helpful in countless situations, but false negatives occur in virtually every type of medical testing, and thyroid tests are no exception. At times the discrepancy is not in the test itself, but in the person's inability to properly metabolize the thyroid hormone circling in the bloodstream.

Because you could have a low thyroid condition that is not detected by standard lab tests, you may have been told that despite your many seemingly hypothyroid symptoms, your thyroid is fine, and urged to go on a different type of medication, such as antidepressants.

Diagnosing thyroid based only on lab tests used to be standard allopathic practice; today more and more medical doctors are recognizing the limitations of standard lab tests for thyroid conditions. These days on some lab tests there is a note below the TSH, T3, and T4 findings, indicating that the American Association of Endocrinologists encourages **taking the larger clinical picture including symptoms into account**. If you have a family history or associated symptoms but "normal" tests, here are some ways you can receive further information.

First, consider **consulting an acupuncturist** who specializes in thyroid care. He or she will be interested in the larger clinical picture, including the ebb and flow of your energy, how well your digestive system functions, any food cravings or addictions you struggle with, the quality and duration of your sleep, and so on. Even more than with many other conditions, the thyroid is highly dependent upon a steady stream of energy. No energy means no life.

The acupuncturist will want to **read your pulses** by pressing his or her fingertips against the radial artery at your wrist, thereby getting a sense of pulse rhythm, frequency, quality, and strength. This **gives information** about what is **internally deficient** in the body.

An ideal pulse is strong and evenly rhythmic, like a smooth, rolling ocean wave. If the pulse is weak, thin, or slow, like an ocean wave that has no force behind it to carry it to shore, or choppy like the small breakers you see on rough seas, this can indicate a potential thyroid imbalance within the body.

The acupuncturist will want to look at your tongue, observing the shape of the tongue, the color of the tongue body, and the color of the tongue coating, as well as whether there are any cracks in the tongue body or teeth marks on the sides of the tongue. An ideal tongue is a healthy rosy pink with a thin white coating, with no cracks or teeth marks.

Go to the mirror and look at your own tongue right now. What do you observe? If you see a pale tongue, teeth marks "scalloping" the sides of the tongue, or a thick tongue coating, these can be signs of Kidney Yang deficiency, which closely corresponds to hypothyroidism. (Conversely, if you see a bright red tongue with no coating and cracks in the tongue body, these can be signs of Kidney Yin deficiency, which closely corresponds to hyperthyroidism.)

Other associated symptoms you might observe within yourself are digestive disturbances, sleeplessness, generalized anxiety, a feeling like you have no energy in reserve, and difficulty bouncing back from exertion or adversity.

Remember that in Acupuncture theory, low thyroid often corresponds to a diagnosis of Kidney Yang deficiency, whereas high thyroid often corresponds to a diagnosis of Kidney Yin deficiency. Thus, the digestive difficulty can occur because Kidney Yang deficiency leads to Spleen Yang deficiency (which causes abdominal pain, loose stools, tiredness after eating, and lack of appetite).

The sleep difficulties can occur because the Kidney Meridian and the Heart Meridian are paired in terms of energy, emotions, and insomnia (the Kidney Meridian represents Water, and the Heart Meridian represents Fire; without the cooling influence of the Kidney Meridian, heat overwhelms the Heart Meridian, causing insomnia). Generalized anxiety and irritation can occur because the Heart Meridian houses the mind, and the Liver Meridian is the seat of the emotions (both of which are dependent upon nourishment from the Kidney Meridian).

The interconnectedness of the Meridians is at the crux of Acupuncture theory. Each piece is critically important to the others. When it is deficient, the others topple like dominos.

Thus, a person could have:

- A Kidney Meridian deficiency from a thyroid condition (lack of energy, feeling of nothing in reserve)
- Which fails to nourish the Heart Meridian (leading to sleeplessness and further exhaustion)
- Which causes a Lung Meridian deficiency (resulting in more grief over one's debilitated health)
- Which leads to a stagnation of the Liver Meridian (manifesting in irritability and hypersensitivity to anxiety-provoking situations)
- That causes a Spleen Meridian deficiency (disrupting the digestive processes, thus not allowing proper utilization of food as body fuel)
- Which ultimately results in further Kidney Meridian deficiency.

If these symptoms—and the unfortunate cycle that creates them—sound at all familiar to you, we have good news: *help is on the way.* Once you have been successful in getting better assistance and information for evaluating a suspected thyroid problem, treatment options become much clearer. I am also happy to speak with you by phone to help you begin taking your steps using the philosophy I have been trained in.

In the following chapters we go into depth on treatment possibilities; keep reading to find specific treatments for your individual challenges.

THE BOTTOM LINE

- The standard TSH test, very useful for severe thyroid problems, is *woefully inadequate* for diagnosing most thyroid conditions.
- **Most people have milder forms of thyroid imbalance**, contributing to a variety of types of psychological disturbance.
- Do not accept TSH testing as your complete thyroid evaluation.
- Any TSH above 3.0 is highly suspicious for thyroid abnormality.
- **Venous blood**, the standard blood drawn from the crook of the arm, is **not as accurate as capillary blood**, drawn from a fingertip.
- **Capillary blood** from a quick finger stick is immediately dried on special filter paper, fixing the specimen so the amount of TSH is stable.
- *Always remember:* you could still be low or high thyroid, **even with normal blood tests**.
- If the test shows positive, you can rely on it. **If the test shows normal or negative, you may rightfully question or explore this further.** Do not be intimidated into abdicating your rights.
- Thyroid is one of the **most inherited of all medical conditions**.
- **Related conditions** are medical situations not considered very serious.
- **Physical signs** are detectable aspects that are not necessarily symptoms, yet could cause a person to complain. Temperature taking can provide an example.
- For your best evaluation, be sure to consider **symptoms, family history, related conditions, and physical signs**. These, in addition to blood or saliva testing, help you achieve a correct diagnosis.
- **A jump start for all types includes** vitamins and minerals, antioxidants, omega oils, and amino acids.
- You can **self-order your saliva testing** at www.CanaryClub.org.
- **Acupuncture** can help balance your symptoms before they escalate.

RECOMMENDED ACTION PLAN

- Know that **you could still have a thyroid imbalance**, even with "normal" results on regular blood tests.

- Choose instead the new and **more accurate panel of finger-stick blood tests**, available at www.CanaryClub.org under "Thyroid Tests."

- Also **take the questionnaire**. Be *very suspicious* for a thyroid diagnosis if you have significant symptoms, family history, or physical signs.

- Begin your ongoing jump start each morning by taking a strong dose* of:

  — Multivitamins (four daily Multigenics)

  — Antioxidants (one daily Oxygenics)

  — Omega oils (one daily Omega-EFA)

  — Amino acids (one scoop BioPure Protein)

  *For more information on our brand recommendations, please see Metagenics on page 279.

PART II

Understand Your Best Treatment

This section presents five of the most common psychological afflictions caused by either high or low thyroid.

Often, people are a mix of these individual mind-types. Still, it can be extremely helpful to begin by addressing the one main way that your thyroid is affecting you.

To use Part II optimally, we recommend that you *focus first on the chapter that most addresses your issues.* **Treating the main issue first will often improve secondary complaints.**

This section reveals five different thyroid treatment plans, each individualized for the particular symptoms needing resolution.

Many practitioners try to treat everyone's thyroid condition with the same medicine; we disagree with this approach. For best results, we recommend that you start with the exact remedies in one of these five treatment plans presented in Chapters 4 through 8. If this treatment proves to be less than fully effective for you, then definitely consider trying a different regimen.

You are entitled to help shape *any* treatment program prescribed to you. Remember that it is your body, and your life.

4

The MOODY Mind-Type
Overcome Depression, Mood Swings, and Negative Thinking

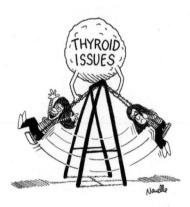

Rosie's Story

Rosie was incredibly depressed. Ever since her husband's premature death, she felt as if life's joy had been snatched from her. She was also gaining weight.

She had likely been depressed for decades. She always had a propensity for hiding out in her bedroom, even as a girl. In her later years, she was simply not available. She made no calls, and rarely spoke. She did not want to have to bother to get dressed, for anyone.

(continued)

When her sons married, she did not attend. In her final years, she insisted that only her sons visit, not their wives. She took little joy in her grandchildren, often appearing eager for them to leave.

Rosie had been diagnosed when young with Hashimoto's thyroid, as was her sister Ann. In later life, when Ann died of cancer, Rosie felt very alone. Her sons had made lives of their own, often traveling. Though she had funds, she did not enjoy travel.

Her doctors tried everything, including thyroid meds, which she clearly needed. Yet nothing helped fully. Occasionally she would feel a bit better, but then would crash right back into depression.

Now we know that a different type of thyroid medication was indicated for her treatment, but we were not treating her then. Rosie, like most thyroid patients, had been given an inactive form of thyroid hormone—in her case, the standard Synthroid brand of T4 (thyroxine)— as the full treatment for her condition. What she needed, however, was some active thyroid hormone, T3 (thyronine), added to the T4.

A simple fix was all that stood between Rosie and her deepening depression.

It only came about near her end, when her niece, a West Coast physician, visited and recognized that her thyroid was out of whack. Rosie was put on a mixture of medicines (the T3/T4 combo) and, actually for the first time in decades, started to feel like her old self.

In Rosie's honor, we beg of you: If people you love seem depressed, consider their thyroid status very carefully, even if they are already on thyroid medicine. Get all the right tests, including a Free T3 level and thyroid antibodies. In addition, make sure they receive a trial of T3 added to their T4, so you can be sure if the thyroid is or is not part of the depression problem.

What's at Stake

Depression is the most common of all mental disorders. According to the World Health Organization (2003: *investing in Mental Health*):

- Up to 450 million people worldwide suffer from mental/behavioral disorders.
- Nearly 1 million people commit suicide every year.

- Four of the six leading causes of disability are due to neuro-psychiatric disorders (depression, alcoholism, schizophrenia, bipolar disorder). (Costa)
- One of every four families has at least one member with a mental disorder. Family members are often the primary caregivers for people with mental problems. The extent of the burden of mental disorders on family members is difficult to assess, but surely it has a significant impact on the family's quality of life.
- In addition to the health and social costs, those suffering from mental illnesses are also victims of human rights violations, stigma, and discrimination, both inside and outside psychiatric institutions.

Additional "Depressing" Facts

- In the United States alone, **depression affects more than 40 million people**. For the years 2003 to 2006, the Centers for Disease Control and Prevention (CDC) reported that the number of people taking an SSRI antidepressant medicine was 17 million.
- Depression is **twice as common in women**, starting at puberty into adulthood. This gender preference and puberty factor are suspiciously similar for thyroid illness. (Westly)
- Even bipolar illness, also known as manic depression, shows a **gender preference for women**, who tend to have lower lows than men. (Harrison)

Better Thyroid Care:
A Hopeful and Easy Fix

What do we really know about thyroid and depression?

Here is a statement from one of the doctors in the field who has been treating both depression and hypothyroidism for more than 25 years. "Low thyroid is one of the main, frequently overlooked and undiagnosed causes of depression. The status of the thyroid gland is often the *key* issue in depression; it *needs* to be addressed and corrected." This physician has also summarized the best research studies and is convinced that close to 40% of depression is caused by the thyroid. (Ross)

Very recent studies have shown that only one out of every three or four patients with depression responds well to antidepressant drugs. This is in sharp contrast to the percentages of success in thyroid treatment. Most all people treated for thyroid imbalance have a favorable response to their thyroid medicine. Thus, thyroid imbalance is more easily and more successfully treated than depression.

Depression is especially hard to treat if the practitioner *thinks* he is treating clinical depression but is actually treating a mental symptom of thyroid imbalance.

> **Thyroid abnormalities do not resolve well when treated with only antidepressants and/or psychotherapy. They resolve best when treated with thyroid medicines.**

If your depression is all or partly a thyroid symptom, you need thyroid treatment and not necessarily antidepressants.

Another reason to be cautious about antidepressants is that they can be harmful in certain cases. In December 2009, the prestigious *Archives of Internal Medicine* published an article written by Jordan Smoller, MD, from Harvard's Massachusetts General Hospital. It concluded that **postmenopausal women taking either a tricyclic antidepressant** (TCA) or a **selective serotonin reuptake inhibitor** (SSRI) appear to **be at increased risk for hemorrhagic and fatal stroke**. This information came from an analysis of the Women's Health Initiative. (WHI study)

Health: The New Bottom Line

Edgar Cayce, considered America's foremost predictor of events, envisioned huge chasms in the Earth's surface around this time, with land formations undergoing transformation. Whether or not that happens physically, it certainly does seem to be happening inside of us, and in our lives.

For anyone out there who is feeling overly sad, overly mad, or even over-the-top overly glad, you may need hormone help.

> **Epidemiology experts conservatively estimate that *one-third of all depressions are directly related to thyroid imbalance*.**

A Groundbreaking Book

Hundreds of scientific articles studying this connection have been marshalled in a groundbreaking book, *The Thyroid Axis and Psychiatric Illness.* (Joffe)

This major review focused on the last 25 years, identifying the connection between thyroid dysfunction and various types of depression. They found so many positive correlations that the mountains of data had to be divided into three different categories:

1. Commonly finding thyroid issues in patients previously diagnosed with depression.
2. Commonly finding depression in patients previously diagnosed with thyroid issues.
3. Beneficial results of thyroid treatment in patients diagnosed with depression.

In all three areas, numerous studies confirm a *strong thyroid-depression link*. What all this means is simple.

> **A significant percentage of people with depression have some degree of thyroid imbalance. Treating the thyroid issue improves the depression.** (Lowe)

If you have depression of any kind, whether mild or severe, *if it is related to thyroid*, as many depressions are, then simple thyroid treatment can be enormously helpful to you.

This is certainly relevant to people with regular depression. It is even more relevant to those with bipolar depression, especially the rapid-cycling type. In treating depression with thyroid hormone, these groups have experienced the most success.

Thyroid-Brain Connections

How could an ordinary and routine gland like the thyroid play such a monumental role?

*   Thyroid hormone has sweeping and profound effects on biological functions of the body's cells and tissues, **particularly in the brain**.
*   In the brain, **thyroid hormone is responsible for controlling the**

rate of synthesis of our key brain chemicals, the neurotransmitters. These include dopamine, serotonin, adrenaline, and noradrenaline.

- These chemicals are **crucial to the brain functions that result in thoughts and feelings.** The most common psychiatric medicines regulate the amount of these neurotransmitters. For instance, Prozac and its numerous cousins, including Paxil, Zoloft, Remeron, Effexor, and Lexapro, etc., are used to increase levels of serotonin available in the brain's synapses for transmission of nerve impulses.

Medical "Mood Drugs"

Prior to the development of these extremely common psychiatric medicines, tricyclic antidepressants were used. These worked by increasing the levels of adrenaline, noradrenaline, and dopamine.

These medicines are called **antidepressants** because of their ability to lighten a depressed mood. Current research reveals:

- According to Irving Kirsch, PhD, professor of psychiatry at the University of Hull in England, **popular antidepressants** are at best weakly effective for relieving symptoms of depression and **do not fully correct disrupted brain chemistry**.
- This revealing new take on the usefulness of antidepressants is thoroughly documented in Dr. Kirsch's new book, *The Emperor's New Drugs.*
- Interestingly, as if in support of Dr. Kirsch, *The Journal of the American Medical Association (JAMA)* featured a study in January 2010 showing that psychoactive drugs are no better than placebos for mild to moderate depression. (Kirsch)
- It should be noted that current antidepressant drugs have a wide variety of chemical structures and effects, but they all work equally well. What does that tell you? (Flora)

   The major overlooked antidepressant, par excellence, is *thyroid hormone,* which really *can* correct disrupted brain chemistry.

Are we saying that low thyroid is the cause of everybody's depressed state? No, of course not.

There are a great many other reasons for depression. Nevertheless, proper thyroid health is of key importance in relation to any discussion of depression, since lack of thyroid hormone is one of the major causes of depression.

Postpartum Mood Disorders

Postpartum depression is one particular kind of depression that is well known to have a *clear medical cause.* It is most often, in reality, a postpartum flare-up of a latent thyroid problem.

Postpartum depression is one type of temporary depression. It can range from mild to severe, with the onset occurring up to 6 months following childbirth. The strong connection of this type of depression to thyroid has been well documented.

Medical researchers, who have carefully studied this, estimate that 80% to 90% of **postpartum depression is actually postpartum thyroiditis**. This situation occurs when an inflammation of thyroid tissue follows an increase in thyroid antibody formation, after the delivery of a baby.

> **Much of postpartum depression is clearly postpartum *thyroid* imbalance.**

Mechanisms for Depression after Birth

During pregnancy, certain immune system activity is reduced so that the immune cells and antibodies will not reject the baby's placenta, which is temporarily grafted onto the inside of the mother's uterus.

After 9 months the situation changes. The baby is pushed out, the placenta releases, and aspects of the immune system that were turned down to prevent early rejection of this graft are now turned back up.

Keep in mind, a graft from another person, in this case a baby to the mother's uterus, is not abided well by the immune system. If later in life this same child wanted to give the mom a skin graft, there may be a rejection of the child's skin by the mom. The immune system rejects what is different.

The baby has different characteristics—half from the father, half from the mother. It is a different person, and the immune system would realize that, then reject that graft. This does not happen in embryonic life because that part of the immune system that would do the rejecting is toned down. But once that returns to normal, it returns with a surge.

This "surge" is akin to power surges that can occasionally occur in your home or office, requiring the protection of a surge protector (in the case of your computer). After being off for a while, the power comes back on, briefly at a higher level than normal. That surge can cause a huge disruption to sensitive electrical equipment.

In a similar fashion, the immune system surges back into action, perhaps at first higher than ordinarily. This surge can result in disruption of the sensitive immune regulatory systems of the body.

It is well documented that within 2 to 6 months after a birth, thyroid problems are *exceedingly common.* This is due to a surge in antibodies that target the thyroid, resulting in noticeable thyroid imbalance. As with many power surges, this disruption is often quite brief.

Surge Protection

Sometimes the surge can cause a change that is not so temporary. A woman experiencing this autoimmune surge might have her thyroid function significantly disrupted. This could last for a few weeks, months, or even years. In some cases, it can be a change that persists until it is diagnosed and treated.

Sometimes the postpartum onset of low thyroid, called hypothyroidism, can last for many years. Sometimes the onset of high thyroid, called hyperthyroidism, can likewise last for a number of years. More often, after a shorter period of time, the hypo- or hyperthyroid condition will then gradually diminish and return to normal.

We are not suggesting that *all* **postpartum depressions are caused by thyroid abnormality.** The scientific fact is that *many of them are.*

The postpartum variety is simply one of many kinds of depression that are also partly thyroid related. A significant percentage of depression in general is determined by how much thyroid hormone is available to the brain. Keeping these hormones flowing is our goal.

Scientific Documentation

How much of everyday depression, now being treated with Prozac or psychotherapy, is actually due to low thyroid? When you read the hypothyroidism literature, the topic of depression is prevalent.

Depression is a major correlate of low thyroid. It is one of the cardinal symptoms of this kind of hormone imbalance. (Hendrick)

- Low mood has been described as part of the hypothyroid picture for well over 100 years. Medical writers began describing adverse mental, emotional, and behavioral effects of untreated hypothyroidism in the late 19th century.
- In 1880, for example, G. H. Savage wrote an article for the *Journal of Mental Science*. The title of the article was "Myxedema and Its Nervous Symptoms." (*Myxedema* was a word for hypothyroidism at that time.) Depression was known, even at that early time, to be a common part of the experience of a hypothyroid person.
- In 1891, G. R. Murray published an article for the *British Medical Journal*, called "Note on the Treatment of Myxedema by Hypodermic Injection of an Extract of the Thyroid Gland of a Sheep." This was one of the early attempts to treat the commonly seen condition of low thyroid, by injecting thyroid glandular from another animal.

Even Earlier History

This glandular maneuver, first described back in 1891 by Western doctors, was known for perhaps a thousand years before that in China. There, doctors treated the condition of low energy, low mood, chilliness, and weight gain with a nutritional remedy called duck neck soup. The entire neck of the duck—including the thyroid gland—was made into a soup and fed to the patient.

This treatment resulted in miraculous improvement for large numbers of patients suffering from this persistent and difficult problem. Just as Murray had discovered, the Chinese doctors had earlier found that people so treated had more energy, less chilliness, less constipation, and also a brighter mood. (For more on Chinese Medicine, be sure to read the section toward the end of each chapter, called "Complementary Healing for Your Best Results.")

For more than a thousand years, doctors have known that treating hypothyroidism improves mood. Indeed, a low mood with depressive behavior has been extensively described as a prominent part of the hypothyroid presentation.

Psychological changes, especially low mood, may be the earliest or most prominent feature of hypothyroidism.

The conversion of T4 into active T3 is diminished in patients who are depressed. This brings up the possibility that in depressed patients there is a "central nervous system hypothyroidism" not showing up as a total-body hypothyroidism on blood tests.

The presence of the right amount of thyroid hormone seems to produce an increase in availability of serotonin in the brain. Some researchers have even suggested that one of the reasons Prozac works so well in some people is that it increases the level of T3 thyroid hormone in key nervous system structures.

Biochemical Advances

Medical science has recently begun to focus in earnest on the biochemistry of depression in relation to thyroid function. Researchers now realize that thyroid is the throttle and manager of brain biochemistry.

Brain effects of hypothyroidism include depression, emotional lability, mental sluggishness, diminished spontaneity, indifference, and self-accusatory ruminations. (Weiner)

The medical literature is replete with documentation of this symptom list. Medical writers describe adverse mental, emotional, and behavioral effects of untreated hypothyroidism. They also describe exceptional improvement in mental symptoms upon thyroid treatment. (Walker)

Not only is depression related to hypothyroidism. The increase in severity of the hypothyroidism is associated with an increase in severity of the depression.

The patient initially may have vague symptoms, such as weakness and lack of interest in life. As the hypothyroidism progresses, there may be complaints of many other symptoms, including trouble concentrating, sluggish thinking, diminished ability to calculate mentally, decreased ability to answer questions, and decreased ability to express oneself.

As the severity progresses, ability for and interest in routine daily tasks diminish further. People become less attentive and responsive to others, lacking concern for their surroundings. They may also lose the capacity for learning and performing new tasks. Their actions and thinking are likely to be slow.

Eventually, there is an increase in drowsiness and lethargy, with progressively lower mood. Sometimes the worsening depressive thoughts can lead to suicide attempts. Profound hypothyroidism, the most extreme, can lead to stupor, and then coma. (Braverman)

Acceptance of the Biochemical View

For several generations, behavioral psychologists and psychoanalysts seemed uninterested in the biochemical reasons for depression. Only more recently have biochemical causes been considered worthy of exploration. Perhaps the reason is that only recently have the actual biochemical mechanisms of depression been better understood. (Smith)

Newer technologies have made such understanding more accessible. The actual mechanism of thyroid hormone action inside the nuclei and mitochondria of cells has been well understood only in the last 20 or 30 years. The same is true for the details of other important brain activity, such as glial cell nourishment, or the biochemistry of long-term memory. (Morton)

Just how common is depression in hypothyroidism? In one study of 100 hypothyroid patients, 60% of them were significantly depressed.

An earlier report described the symptom of depression in 23% of patients with a mildly low metabolism. This means that even mild hypothyroidism can cause significant depression.

Making the Connection

These reports above were of *thyroid patients who seemed depressed*. What about psychiatric patients with low mood? How many certifiably depressed people with no outward hint of thyroid would have a significant thyroid problem if you tested carefully for it?

In one study, researchers have reported that figure to be 25%. (Loosen)

The study utilized the extra-accurate thyrotropin-releasing hormone (TRH) test. This technology is highly dependable, but also very costly. It is not used often in general thyroid care outside of university settings. It does, however, help to point out the extent of hypothyroidism hidden in depressed populations.

Once again, in depressed people with no overt signs or physical symptoms of hypothyroidism, 25% had a hidden thyroid dysfunction. What do you suppose would be the percentage in a population of depressed people *who also have physical symptoms* of fatigue, overweight, chilliness, constipation, excessive hair loss, or dry skin and cracking nails? Here, the incidence of diagnosable hypothyroidism is even greater.

Consider this example: in a study of patients with *severe* depression, the amount of hypothyroidism was found to be up to 50%. In another study, this time of *refractory* depression (resistant to antidepressant treatment), 90% had clinical indications of hypothyroidism. Also, and more important, **the administration of thyroid hormone relieved most of the patients' depression**. (Gewirtz)

One big problem in this research is the inadequacy of the regular thyroid tests (T4, TSH). These tests are often not fully reliable in detecting subtle hypothyroidism in depressed patients. Patients may need better testing—including *Free T3* levels and *thyroid antibodies*—to be diagnosed accurately.

What if the better tests are still normal, but patient and practitioner remain suspicious for thyroid imbalance? Then a TRH determination is the next step, though costly. A trial of thyroid treatment is the final arbiter even though a more sensitive panel of tests reveals more of the depressed people who actually have treatable thyroid imbalance. (Loosen)

Mechanisms That Impact Mood

If depression and hypothyroidism are causally linked, what are some of the actual biochemical mechanisms? Is it simply that low thyroid causes sluggish brain function and that sluggish brain function results in depression? While this may be a convenient way to understand the situation, a more detailed explanation can be useful.

- **Several studies have shown that low levels of thyroid hormone result in less secretion of noradrenaline.** Less of this neurotransmitter in the brain stem and the limbic area results in depression. (Nichols)

- **Another mechanism is a decrease in the beta-adrenaline receptors.** In thyroid deficiency, the density of these hormone receptors on the cell membranes decreases. This decrease results in a dominance of the alpha-adrenaline receptors. The end result here is a slowing of intracellular metabolic process. (Gross)

This **metabolic slowing** explains why most hypothyroid patients are found to be cool and sluggish, with low blood pressure, *and appear to have a very low mood*. It is as if these people have a decrease in sympathetic nervous system function at the level of brain cell receptors. (Gross)

Change in **type and density of receptor sites** is a significant aspect of the hypothyroidism-depression connection, helping to explain the success of psychiatrists in using thyroid hormone to augment their psychotropic medicines. Numerous studies demonstrate that T3 heightens nerve tissue response to antidepressants, mostly likely due to a change in the receptor density. Even mild hypothyroidism, falsely within the normal range on regular lab tests, can affect brain tissue so as to invite depression. (Prange)

Serotonin Receptors

Serotonin levels may also interact with thyroid hormone to cause or contribute to depression.

- The neurotransmitter *serotonin* is of key importance in emotional states, specifically depression. Serotonin-related fibers from the brain stem go to brain regions that control many different mood-related behaviors.

- **The treatment for depression has in recent years focused on trying to intensify serotonin function.** Thyroid hormone plays a key role in the regulation of serotonin levels. (Schwark)

- Serotonin receptors, quite abundant in the limbic areas of the brain, are found to be highly involved in depression. These same areas of the brain also have a high level of gene expression for three different types of thyroid hormone receptors.

- Researchers have concluded that there is a neuro-modulation link between the thyroid system and serotonin receptors in the limbic region of the brain. (Tejani-Butt)

This means that decreased serotonin activity contributes to the observed depression in hypothyroid patients.

MAO Inhibitors

Another mechanism whereby low thyroid contributes to or causes depression is related to the monoamine oxidase arena. MAO, as it is abbreviated, is the enzyme that helps quickly deactivate the neurotransmitters adrenaline and noradrenaline after they perform their function in the synapses.

MAO is produced in the tiny intracellular powerhouses called mitochondria. The enzymatic process deactivates the neurotransmitter by a maneuver called deamination. Blocking this process allows more neurotransmitter to be available to influence the synapse. The result of more neurotransmitter activity is a brighter mood.

Some years ago, a whole category of MAO-inhibiting antidepressants grew out of this research. These were extremely effective and useful mood elevators, except for some very bothersome side effects. Today they are much less popular than the SSRI category, which includes Prozac.

When thyroid is low, MAO activity increases. This increased activity reduces the quantity of noradrenaline and adrenaline available at the synapse. That reduces the adrenergic drive, which then leads to depression.

Adding thyroid hormone reverses the above process, and depression is lifted. This thyroid connection is so critical that it led some researchers to imagine that thyroid hormone might be an inducible MAO inhibitor itself, suggesting that thyroid hormone itself is an antidepressant. (Assad)

It is known that the administration of thyroid hormone is accompanied by a decrease in MAO activity. The mechanism proposed is that thyroid hormone controls the level of the MAO inhibitory modulator, by regulating mitochondrial MAO activity, via thyroid hormone's control over gene induction. To state this a bit more simply:

Thyroid hormone works really well for depression.

This line of reasoning has led a number of researchers to conclude that when there is depression due to thyroid-related low levels of serotonin or noradrenaline, the proper treatment is to give thyroid hormone to the patient, rather than antidepressants.

It is well known that depressed hypothyroid patients respond well to their thyroid hormone therapy. It is often accompanied by complete or partial relief of the depression.

Thyroid Hormone as an Antidepressant

Much of the research in this area has focused on combining thyroid hormone with an antidepressant. Less common has been the idea of using thyroid hormone itself, *alone*, as an antidepressant. (Goodwin)

> **The therapeutic goal of treating hypothyroidism by bringing the TSH level into the normal range does not relieve all of the symptoms for many patients.**

Many individuals do not get relief until there is enough medication given to bring the TSH level down to the low-normal range, or even slightly **below normal** range. This method of using thyroid hormone is popular with a number of doctors today, including many in the academic arena, but not yet in the mainstream.

> **It should be noted that many people's depression does not resolve until the dose of thyroid is raised so TSH levels become low-normal or actually go into the low range.** (Surks)

Conversely, more forward-looking researchers consider that thyroid hormone might relieve severe depression, even when there is no clear evidence of hypothyroidism. This actual process has been observed in "drug-resistant depression" and in women.

What's clear is that various depression treatments have definite effects on thyroid function and testing. For example, lithium, a medicine for manic depression, has been extensively studied for adversely affecting TSH levels and thyroid hormone levels. Other antidepressant medicines (including some of the antiseizure medicines that are sometimes used to treat depression) have effects on thyroid tests as well, although their effect on underlying thyroid function is less clear than in the case of lithium.

To review:

- There is a definite place for the use of thyroid hormones, particularly T3 and also T4, in treatment of depression. (Prange, Wilson)
- These hormones have been shown to be **valuable** in converting **patients who are nonresponsive to antidepressant treatment** into more responsive patients. (Coppen)

- In addition, thyroid **accelerates response to antidepressant treatment** for many, even when antidepresssants are already partially successful. (Wheathley, Thase)
- The overall conclusion we are able to reach is that thyroid hormone plays an important part in the regulation of mood and is closely involved in the actual process of depression.
- It is also clear that these correlations and benefits have been frequently overlooked and are currently under-utilized in research and treatment.
- Several studies have confirmed using **small amounts of T3**, active thyroid hormone, to **potentiate response to antidepressants** in people who were previously nonresponsive to them. (Whybrow)
- The consistent finding was that approximately half of the patients nonresponsive to certain antidepressants will become responsive to them within 2 to 3 weeks after the addition of 25 to 50 mcg of T3 to their previous antidepressant regimen. (Goodwin, Schwarcz)

Our Treatment Recommendations

Below we have listed specific substances that have been shown to improve the conditions we address in each chapter.

Rosemary

For people challenged with sluggish brain function due to thyroid imbalance, one of the best natural over-the-counter remedies available without a prescription is a medicinal form of the herb rosemary.

Ideal is a standardized leaf extract of 80 to 100 mg per day. This innocuous-sounding item has within it a crucial ingredient for thyroid function. It is a source of carnosic acid, a key contributor to the ability of thyroid to attach itself to the DNA molecule, enabling it to read the "Book of Life."

Rosemary just happens to be one handy and inexpensive source of this key nutritional item. Carnosic acid is crucial for thyroid hormone to be able to do its magic inside the nuclei of our cells. But it cannot do this important work alone. The process is called hetero-dimerization, which requires another common yet crucial ingredient: vitamin D.

Vitamin D

You may have heard that vitamin D has been elevated in status from a mere vitamin to an actual "co-hormone." One of its important uses in the body is to join carnosic acid in allowing the thyroid hormone molecule to form an active complex around the DNA molecule, so that DNA instructions can be accessed.

> **Vitamin D, in the presence of *carnosic acid*, allows thyroid hormone to work properly.**

You may imagine that vitamin D is readily available, since sunshine on our skin seems to help with this manufacturing job. However, vitamin D is often in short supply for far too many people, especially in those who are depressed.

People with low energy and depression do not get out in the sun as much as others. They also do not eat as sensibly and properly as they should. Even if they take multivitamins, **they may not absorb the vitamin D component because of sluggish intestinal function and the poor absorption so common in sluggish metabolism.**

Perhaps the biggest reason that people are deficient in vitamin D is that the RDA (recommended daily allowance) for this nutrient was put at too low a level. In the 1940s and 1950s, when the original research was being conducted, the National Science Foundation, with the help of other government agencies, set the RDA at 400 international units (IU). As it turns out, people seem to need closer to 4,000 IU of vitamin D per day, especially those challenged with depression.

Excellent versions of this important nutrient are D_3 1000, containing 1,000 IU of vitamin D, and Iso D_3, containing 2,000 IU of vitamin D. Both of these are from Metagenics, Inc., a company that's decades old and doctor trusted.

Multivitamins

In addition to adding rosemary and vitamin D, it is important for Moody mind-types to make sure they take *every day* a very strong, very complete multivitamin with minerals.

After long periods of time with sluggish absorption, a wide array of nutritional deficiencies can manifest.

An effective vitamin supplement intervention can help to overcome this lack, paving the way for more robust metabolism.

Some of the best examples of full-range multivitamins are Wellness Essentials by Metagenics and ActivEssentials by Xymogen. These products include not only vitamins and minerals but also special antioxidants and omega oils (see pages 279–280).

Coenzyme Q_{10}

A particular nutrient available at vitamin stores that is of great benefit to Moody mind-types is coenzyme Q_{10}. Sometimes called simply CoQ_{10}, it is often sold as either a 30-mg or 100-mg pill. We recommend this latter amount as a daily dosage for the Moody mind-types. It energizes while also supporting brain health and neurological performance. It seems to stabilize the cell membrane.

An especially good version of this nutrient is called CoQ-10 ST-100, which is a stabilized and highly absorbable form, mixed with vitamin E and beta-carotene, produced by Metagenics, Inc. Qec 100 is the Xymogen version, designed to promote even better absorption than dry powder versions of this product. Main benefits seem to be activation of the Krebs cycle (energy production system) (see pages 279–280).

5-HTP

In addition to improving your thyroid function to help improve mood, you can utilize certain nutritional substances that inspire this process. One of the most crucial needs of a depressed person is to get more serotonin.

The chemical precursor that becomes serotonin in your body is available at every health food and vitamin store—it's called 5-HTP.

The name stands for 5-hydroxytryptophan. This and its relative, L-tryptophan, help to increase the amount of serotonin available to the brain.

One note of caution: people taking prescription antidepressants must be very careful about also taking serotonin precursors. They are best used instead of the antidepressant—after finishing the antidepressant, or before trying, which is what we suggest. Start with two 500 mg capsules daily.

Do *not* ingest 5-HTP for serotonin boosting while also taking antidepressant drugs.

Tryptophan products were used in the field of psychiatry as actual antidepressants, until they were taken off the market in 1989, due to an unfortunate manufacturing contaminant that caused illness (which had nothing to do with the effect or side effects of tryptophan itself). Oddly enough, this unfortunate incident seems to have occurred around the time that Prozac was being released to the market.

St. John's Wort

The use of the herbal medicine St. John's wort in psychiatry is well documented and researched. Despite its odd name, it is an herbal medicine that has very strong benefits for people struggling with low mood—and it has very few side effects. It is also quite inexpensive, especially as compared to SSRIs.

When coupled with a good thyroid program, the hypericum ingredient of St. John's wort can be as useful as many of the prescription antidepressants used by today's practitioners.

An exceptionally useful version of this herb combines it with several co-factors for better delivery and function; it is called St. John's Wort with Folate and B_{12}. This is a successful mood support formula from Metagenics, Inc., containing 450 mg of the flowering top extract. *Hypericum perforatum* is standardized to 0.3%, and the Hypericin component to 3.0%, amounts shown in research to be quite helpful (see page 279).

SAM-e

This well-researched, over-the-counter nutritional supplement is sometimes recommended by psychiatrists for depression. It has other uses, but its effect on depression is usually quite beneficial, without side effects. Its main drawback is that it is more costly than most nutritional supplements, but it is still less expensive than most SSRI antidepressants. Compared with the average nutritional supplement sold in vitamin stores, SAM-e has a wealth of experimental and clinical data supporting its use.

It generally comes in either 200 or 400 mg. We recommend starting with 200 mg each day, which often can lift mood. If further benefit is needed, try 400 mg daily.

Prescription Medicines

In light of recent findings from the psychiatric community about the benefit of T3 thyroid hormone, it is of interest to anybody with low thyroid who has some depression symptoms to . . .

Make sure you are taking some T3 as part of your thyroid treatment.

Today most people with thyroid conditions are being treated with T4 alone. This includes the large number of hypothyroid patients who have some symptoms of depression that they wish could be alleviated.

A sensible approach, especially because straight T3 can sometimes be too excitatory, would be to **use T3 in the form of desiccated thyroid**. This was the original thyroid medicine for many years (remember duck neck soup?), until it became possible to synthesize the supposed active ingredients, T3 and T4, in the laboratory. Many people improve after adding desiccated thyroid to their program.

Desiccated Thyroid

Desiccated thyroid is a freeze-dried, standardized-strength *animal gland* product. It is used across the world, but it has taken a backseat in latter years to the newer and questionably "better" synthetics.

For many depressed people with extra-sluggish metabolic function, straight thyroxine is not the right choice, even though it is the most often prescribed.

In many cases, the easiest and best approach would be to use desiccated thyroid. This is a combination of T3 and T4 in a natural ratio that would be especially beneficial to depressed people.

The amount of T3 in desiccated thyroids is usually quite sufficient for improving the neurochemical balance in most depressed patients. The natural approach combines T3 and T4, with T1 and T2 (additional thyroid gland factors), and thyrocalcitonin, along with a variety of other items that are not easily measured. This seems to provide a smooth and appropriate boost for sluggish metabolism, especially in the brain.

How to Get Started

As in all thyroid treatment options, the best course of treatment is to **start low** with the amount of the medicine, in this case desiccated thyroid, and **then slowly titrate upward** until the appropriate clinical response is met—in other words until the patient becomes less depressed and is feeling better.

Start low, and go slow.

At our clinic we generally start with a half grain of desiccated thyroid, once a day in the morning. After a period of 3 to 4 weeks, the response is evaluated and the dose is increased to 1 grain. Again, after 3 to 4 weeks, the dose can be increased to 1.5 grains, and perhaps even higher, continuing in this progression as needed.

Many people do quite well with 1 or 2 grains of desiccated thyroid. Some patients, however, have required 3 or 4 grains. These higher levels are utilized *only after a prolonged time at the lower levels,* to ensure proper equilibration for the desired effect. Usually a period of a couple of months of upward titration occurs before choosing the higher doses.

Desiccated thyroid, commonly called Armour, at various times has been in short supply, with one or all strengths of pills being hard to locate. We believe this is because an animal gland is not as profitable to manufacture and sell as patent medicines, such as Synthroid.

We remain concerned when pharmaceutical houses can manipulate the market on such a crucial health issue, affecting so many.

The manufacturing of Armour desiccated thyroid in the United States appears to have passed from one company to another since the Armour (meat packing) Company sold its medicine division. Another company is now making a desiccated thyroid product called Nature-Throid. Still another company in the United States makes a good product called Proloid, although this is earmarked for use only in other countries.

No matter what brand or form, desiccated products have been found to be very useful at our clinic. Other doctors have suggested that the use of synthetic thyroid is preferred for *all* patients. To us, this is absurd!

There is no one best type of thyroid medicine for all patients.

We can understand why the largest HMO in this country wanted every thyroid patient to receive the synthetic brand of thyroxine called Levothroid. Now they know that some people do much better on desiccated thyroid than on Levothroid, and—to their credit—Kaiser Foundation is beginning to allow people to have this desiccated product when the synthetic has proven unsuccessful for the patient.

Desiccated thyroid can be purchased by prescription from a pharmacy, in increments of 0.5-grain or 0.25-grain pills. When the proper dose is reached, say 1.5 grains, such a dosage size exists as a single pill of the brand name Armour. Nature-Throid and Wes-Throid come as either 0.5-, 1-, or 2-grain pills.

How Best to Monitor Your Medicines

The completion of your upward titration, and arrival at an ongoing dose, is reached when there is full relief of symptoms. In addition, blood tests should show normal T3 and T4 levels.

Most practitioners will look mainly at your TSH test results, rather than looking at symptoms, or at the actual levels of thyroid hormone.

We recommend a thorough evaluation to help you arrive at optimal thyroid levels.

Consider symptoms, physical signs, and other thyroid tests—not just TSH.

Many people will be advised to stop their upward titration when the test results, especially TSH, reach normal range. At our clinic, we have found that many thyroid patients do not feel or perform at their best until they have taken an amount of medicine that results in the TSH being below the normal range. Remember, more medicine results in a lower TSH.

Taking an amount of medicine that results in a lower-than-normal TSH is a standard medical procedure, used in many hospitals and clinics, especially research hospitals with treatment of thyroid after cancer treatment.

You do not need to have thyroid cancer to benefit from TSH suppression therapy if it is indicated. Someone not feeling like her old self, not 100%, should have the opportunity to try a higher dose of thyroid medicine than would simply result in a normal TSH test.

A strong dose of medicine that has a person feeling good for the first time in years might result in a TSH level below the normal range; this is fine.

The main problem with too much thyroid hormone is an excessive pushing of the metabolism into "hyper-drive." When this happens, you will generally know. **People overmedicated with thyroid hormone feel like they have had way too much coffee.** They feel hyped up, shaky, and too warm; have too rapid a heart rate and high blood pressure; are too tense in muscles; and have new onset of insomnia coinciding with the higher dosage of thyroid meds.

If you do not have these symptoms, it is unlikely that you are overmedicated with thyroid. Doctors who do not have full experience with hundreds of thyroid patients might tell you, "Oh, you're on too much medicine, even though you don't feel like you're on too much. The TSH test tells us so."

You are *not* overmedicated if you are actually, finally, feeling better at the higher doses.

We have witnessed this over and over in our patients, where they are feeling better than they have in years, but when they see their doctor, he or she tells them their TSH results show they are on too high a dose. So they are taken down in replacement, start feeling worse again, and soon need to be seen again in our clinic, where we have to increase their dosage to get them back to the progress they had made previously.

Blind obedience to one overrated blood test is not good medical care.

Long-Term Management of Your Protocol

Once you have reached a satisfactory dose of thyroid hormone, you may be able to stay at this dose for years. People remain at the same dose that was initially successful for as long as it continues to be a successful dose for them. Doctors who have spent a lot of time with thyroid patients see them in basically two categories:

1. Some, once they have reached a satisfying regimen, find that their body is stable, and they maintain ongoing improvement.

2. Others, however, have more trouble. For them, finding the optimal dose is always like shooting at a moving target. It is common for these people to have mid-course corrections in their dose levels, needed perhaps every 3 to 6 months. Their bodies seem to have some internal fluctuation that results in their needing higher doses at some times, lower at others. It is fine for doctors and these patients to be attuned to these changing needs.

After being on thyroid meds for a year or two, it is a perfectly appropriate question to consider whether or not you can go off thyroid medicine. The answer is yes for *some* people. The way this can work is to go off the medicine even more slowly than your original tapering-up phase. Then see if being off medicine sustains the improvement that was gained being on meds. Be off your meds 100 days before deciding.

This works for certain people. Those who have some healing over these months or years on thyroid medicine can often return to a life without prescription thyroid pills. They may elect instead to take natural remedies mentioned above for their long-term benefit.

Many others, however, are not able to enjoy life nearly as well, or feel nearly as good, off thyroid medicine. They may try going off and find that they really do need it. They may never even try to go off, sensing that they still need it.

How does a person—or practitioner—know that the person needs to stay on thyroid medicine long term?

- If the thyroid condition was **severe** to start with.
- If the **antibody levels were very high**.
- If there was a **special reason that the thyroid was ill-functioning** (surgery on neck or thyroid area, whiplash or other auto injury resulting in neck trauma, or a very strong family history of severe thyroid problems).

This person is likely to need thyroid medicine on an ongoing basis.

Because of the difficulty in deciding which of these camps you could be in, most doctors have adopted the general rule of "once you start thyroid medicine, you stay on it forever." This rule of thumb is handy for doctors, but not fair to patients.

It leaves many people continuing to take thyroid medicines long after they need to do so. Rather than have someone who needs thyroid medicine stop taking it prematurely, the medical recommendation seems to be that everyone stay on it forever.

If you can monitor this situation closely and be aware of the many physical and mental symptoms of inadequately treated low thyroid, then you can safely try gradual thyroid medicine reduction.

Many have the misconception that taking thyroid medicine can make you need it forever. Although some situations are like this in our bodies, thyroid is not one of them.

Whether or not you need thyroid medicine forever has nothing to do with whether you take it for a while. As we said previously, the people who need it forever due to their internal chemistry simply need it forever. Other people have thyroid abnormality that is not too severe. These might well benefit from taking thyroid for a year, then slowing it down. It may also come then go at various times.

Just remember that desiccated thyroid medicine is still one of the best kinds of thyroid for certain people, in certain situations, because it has naturally occurring amounts of T3 and T4, along with T1 and T2, which recent research suggests are also bioactive and helpful to us. Plus, it is generally less costly when compared with synthetic thyroid.

The challenge is that there is a **medical bias**, perhaps inspired by the synthetic patent medicine drugmakers. Just because it is natural does not make it inherently better for you, just as it does not make it worse for you.

> Many people, especially those who are depressed, have had *exceptionally* good results using this animal glandular form of thyroid.

But now for something even more exceptional:

> Any medical program can be improved in effectiveness, with reduced side effects, by the addition of the exquisite overall systemic balancing using acupuncture.

Complementary Healing for Your Best Results

By Georjana Shames, LAc

Interestingly, in writing this book, Drs. Richard and Karilee Shames identified five major categories to help conceptualize different aspects of thyroid mental health. They distilled this view into short descriptive words: *moody, edgy, foggy, sleepy,* and *needy.* At that point they consulted me in terms of what an acupuncturist would say about these five categories.

I was amazed, because in fact these five categories beautifully relate to the classic Acupuncture structure of the Five Elements Theory. For thousands upon thousands of years, the philosophy governing Acupuncture practice has been borne of the Five Elements: Fire, Earth, Metal, Water, and Wood.

Each of these elements signifies a particular acupuncture meridian, such as Heart (Fire), Spleen (Earth), Lung (Metal), Kidney (Water), and Liver (Wood). Remarkably, these meridians closely fit the categories of Moody, Edgy, and so on. Here we see a perfect intersection of East-West integrative medicine.

Let us begin with Moody, which would in this representation fit the Heart Meridian. Remember that in Chinese Medicine the Heart Meridian houses the Mind. This, of course, is responsible for **clear, analytical thinking**. Yet in addition to that, apart from the mental activity aspect, the Mind also affects the emotional state.

- If the Heart is strong, the Mind will also be strong, and the person will be happy.
- If the Heart is weak, the Mind lacks vitality. The person will be sad or depressed, in low spirits.
- If the Heart is in an excess condition, the Mind will be affected. The person may display symptoms of mental illness, such as bipolar.

Of course, this is an oversimplification, as a person's emotional state is related to all the other organs as well. (Maciocia)

Thus, according to ancient Acupuncture understanding, the best treatment approach for a Moody type of person (especially one who is low in thyroid) would be supporting the Heart Meridian with acupuncture points, herbal remedies, dietetic suggestions, and lifestyle guidance.

Acupuncture, the actual insertion of needles, should be performed only by a licensed practitioner. Ideally, you would see a trusted and compassionate acupuncturist who can assist you in maintaining emotional balance.

If, however, you would like to learn techniques for self-care to augment your acupuncture sessions, or if you have not yet found the perfect practitioner, here are *acupressure* points you can press on yourself to get started in the right direction.

CARING FOR YOURSELF

- Locate a spot on the inner wrist about 2 inches toward the elbow from the wrist crease, between the two middle tendons (called Pericardium 6). Press here whenever you feel overwhelmed by sadness. This point strengthens the Heart Meridian and pacifies the Mind.
- Locate the tender spot near the ankle about 3 inches directly above the medial malleolus, that prominent bone of the inner ankle. Massage this point (called Spleen 6) for long-standing depression and mood swings. **Note: Do not press this point if you are pregnant.**

RECIPES AND REMEDIES

Here is a wonderful combination of herbs and foods in a recipe for the Heart Meridian type of thyroid imbalance. This rice pudding (called *congee*) nourishes the Heart and soothes the Mind, helping to alleviate mood swings and depression. Some of the items can be found at your regular grocery store, while others will be readily available at an Asian market.

- Begin by simmering 1 cup of brown rice in 6 cups of water, adding 1 cup of wheat kernels, 10 Chinese dates (jujubes), and 2 ounces of sliced licorice root.
- Simmer for 1 hour, stirring often, and possibly adding some shredded chicken or beef in the last half hour.
- Serve warm, remembering to remove the cooked licorice slices and discard them, and be careful not to eat or bite down on the date pits. This recipe will last for multiple servings. Eat once per day for 2 weeks to see if your mood improves.

LIFESTYLE LIFTS

When it comes to lifestyle, the Heart Meridian type of moodiness responds well to gentle exercise, mindfulness relaxation, and one or more of the following:

- Walk at least once daily for 20 minutes to invigorate the circulation and relieve stress, plus take an additional walk anytime during the day or evening if you notice mood swings coming on.
- Remove yourself from a stressful situation, even briefly, to break the cycle.
- Consider also listening to some mindful relaxation audio when the depression hits. The audio and books of Pema Chödrön, such as *When Things Fall Apart: Heart Advice for Difficult Times* and *Choosing a Fresh Alternative,* are excellent choices. (You can purchase her books and tapes at www.shambhala.org/teachers/pema/bookstore2.php.)
- Laugh. It does a body good and lightens your load on the journey to greater health.

THE BOTTOM LINE

- **A definite link exists between depression and thyroid.** It was originally described more than 100 years ago and has been repeatedly confirmed by numerous investigators over the last 50 years. Recent studies are further expanding this earlier work.
- A **lack of thyroid hormone causes decreased** density of beta-adrenaline **neurotransmitter receptors** in brain cell membranes. One effect of a decrease in these neurotransmitter receptors is depression.
- When tested carefully, depressed patients often reveal **low thyroid** as an underlying **major player** in the **depression** issue.
- **Everyone with depression should be evaluated carefully for thyroid imbalance.** This evaluation should include not just the standard TSH and T4 levels, but also Free T3 and *both* thyroid antibody tests.
- If the above **testing is normal**, but there is **a clear family history of thyroid**, the practitioner should do the more definitive TRH test, or simply provide the patient with a trial of prescription thyroid hormone pills. It can take a few weeks to notice the effects of thyroid medicine.
- Patients with depression and hypothyroidism experience **improvement in their depression when thyroid medicine is added** to their regimen.
- Combining thyroid hormone with an antidepressant (called augmen-tation) is effective in perhaps 50% of people not benefited by antidepressants alone.

- In the brain, **thyroid hormone is responsible for controlling the rate of synthesis of our key brain chemicals**, the neurotransmitters. These include dopamine, serotonin, adrenaline, and noradrenaline.
- Much postpartum depression is postpartum *thyroid* imbalance.
- **Psychological changes**, especially low mood, may be the earliest or most prominent **feature of hypothyroidism**.
- Change in **type and density of receptor sites** is a significant aspect of the hypothyroidism-depression connection.
- There are many **natural products** that can help to **boost thyroid** function, including rosemary, vitamin D, good multivitamins, St. John's wort, SAM-e, coenzyme Q_{10}, and 5-HTP (see page 279).
- Make sure you are taking **some T3** as part of your thyroid treatment. One of the best ways to do this is to take desiccated glandular thyroid, such as Armour or Nature-Throid, as your medicine choice.
- When titrating upward or down on thyroid, **start low and go slow**.
- There is no one best type of thyroid medicine for all patients.
- To help you arrive at optimal thyroid levels, consider symptoms, physical signs, and other thyroid testing—not just TSH.
- Do not believe that you are overmedicated if you are actually, finally, feeling better at the higher doses. Listen to your body!
- Any program can be enhanced using integrative therapies, such as acupuncture, to ensure a smooth recovery.

RECOMMENDED ACTION PLAN

- For over-the-counter treatment of thyroid-related depression, start with two pills daily of a thyroid booster containing standardized rosemary extract (like Thyrosol, from Metagenics).
- Also add two pills daily of a **high-quality vitamin D** (such as D_3 1000, from Metagenics).
- If these measures are not fully helpful, add to your jump start a **stepwise increasing trial of prescription desiccated thyroid**, such as Armour or Nature-Throid, from a qualified practitioner.

The EDGY Mind-Type

Reduce Anxiety, Panic, Irritability, Anger, and Rage

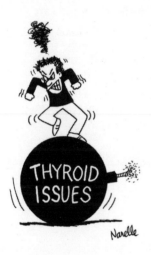

Flo's Story

She surely loved her children and meant well in her heart. Yet on most days she was raging. She just couldn't seem to help herself; a constant war zone surrounded and trailed her. It had been her family legacy, that unrestrained rage; she came by it legitimately.

(continued)

Her children learned when young to scatter, hiding in the obscure caverns of their very disjointed home. Her anxiety was contagious. She seemed to truly lack what many mothers had, a sense of stability and calm, yet she had an amazing strength of her own. She was fierce and angry, Vesuvius spewing, much of the time. Yet she was filled with an amazing love.

A beautiful girl in her younger years, Flo always had that spark that attracted men. Unfortunately, it later grew into a flame, burning those around her. With a houseful of kids, it didn't get any better. Flo was an explosion waiting to happen, a train wreck in slow-mo. Normally, she appeared anxious and nervous, perhaps from a very young age, when fears dominated her waking moments.

Could all those painful years raising her children have been different? What if she had actually received **optimal thyroid care** early on?

Thankfully, there is a happy ending to this story. In later years, Flo is improved. She is on thyroid pills and has a solid calmness about her. It is uncertain that she would have mellowed with age anyway.

What definitely inspired this change was better thyroid care. Fixing her thyroid allowed her to create and enjoy a better life!

Your Way Out: Stop Being a "Mess on Stress"

Flo, in the story above, was—like many of us—a "mess on stress." Since the apple doesn't fall far from the tree, family behaviors are likely to continue from one generation to the next unchanged, unless we live more consciously, committed to improving our familial-behavioral inheritance.

Those from troubled backgrounds have higher hurdles to clear in behaving more "normally." It is a process, and we are always works in progress.

First, Baby Steps

We need to find that balance between *unconscious repetition* (in which we continue dysfunctional patterns, often when tired or stressed) **and** *blaming ourselves* for repeating harmful, unpleasant familial behaviors. Most of us, as humans, are likely to repeat patterns at times; it is our nature. In other words:

> Take the best and leave the rest.
> Forgiveness is our fertile nest.
> Life is not always just a test—
> Still, always do your best.
> Forgive (when you can)
> Forget when you must,
> Listen to your spirit,
> Use caution with your trust.

New Directions

The good news is that we can learn, through time and tedious hard work, to behave differently. This section actually provides "new directions," not only for your health but also for your life. In our expanded view, life and health are not separate. Health is what guides and informs our life.

We can become the person we want to be, rather than being defined by old "family" rules. We can change the way we think, act, and behave, especially as we gain optimal metabolism.

We hope to continue to inspire you to attain wholeness, which is wellness, without which our lives have little joy. Joy is the candle that lights our days.

It is imperative for us all to learn to take charge of our lives. Those of us who grew up in dysfunctional homes must take exceptional care of ourselves. Since many out-of-control people have hormonal imbalance, this can be a way *out* of the shame, blame, and rage that may have plagued our families for generations. It is up to us, here and now, to make it better.

One crucial place to start is in minimizing our stressors. Stop stressing. This is easier than you may imagine, once you do it, and of enormous value.

Erica's Story

Erica seems to pride herself on her ability to withstand terrible pressure and pain; at times it seems she fights Nature herself.

In many ways Erica is deeply connected to the Earth. Yet, there is this overbearing part of her, muscling its way through her stressful life, challenging and defying and rebutting and using the mind, so very quickly, leaving her unable to hear the heart and words of others.

Her excuse? There are many: she's exhausted. She has to stay focused on the crisis at hand. She bought decaf instead of regular by mistake. There's more on her plate than she can handle. Her husband is not able to help enough. And so on.

What will it take for her to recognize that she is the creator of her own out-of-control life? What will finally allow her to put her armor down, to listen carefully when others speak, without the perceived need for continuous self-defense?

She disdains direct feedback, all the while saying she knows it comes from Love. She seems to want and need help, yet snaps at the hand that seeks to feed her, most often when she is reminded of how her process has gotten her into trouble in the past.

In those moments of blinding response, she is not centered. She is moving too quickly to witness her life. She may never have known, or must have forgotten, the power of a life lived in balance. Sadly, she seems not to want to be reminded.

Where to Start?

We must **minimize the obvious sources of stress in our lives**. Stress is killing us and the joy in our families. Stress melts us down, fries our brains, and leaves us feeling wasted.

Some people seem to thrive on stress, as if it feeds an inner thirst. The rest of us, the majority, are a mess on stress. Even those who seem to like being on stress hormones will crash surprisingly hard when they do finally crash.

Learning to manage our stress levels is every bit as important as learning to manage our finances, our diet, and our energy.

We each need to understand how stress personally impacts our health and learn to put a lid on situations that are simply not healthy for us. Since we see so many women in our practice, we can assure you that it appears to be most challenging at this time for women.

Women's work in today's world is, by its very nature, overwhelming at times. Most women, as mothers, try too hard and work too much. Whereas mothers in the era we matured in (the 1950s) were expected to stay at home and raise their kids, today's moms don't have that luxury. Instead, most are expected to work—and to clean—*and* to raise their kids. Not to mention being enticing to their partners on top of it all.

> **Perfection is the poison driving us to do too much today; insanity is the result.**

All these time-saving devices were supposed to give us better lives; yet here we are, more trapped than ever, with growing demands.

An Especially Vexing Problem for Women

Women often multitask more than men, and many of us have taken great pride in being able to do so. However, multitasking is turning us all into nervous wrecks. Just because we *can* do something does not mean it is worth doing, or even a good idea.

> **We must learn to live with *less stress*. Avoid as many sources of stress as you possibly can.**

As simple as this may sound, most women are plagued by excessive work, excessive worry, and excessive exhaustion. Something has to give; we recommend you let it be those aspects of your life that you find draining.

If we humans were in better shape, we might still be able to plow on, doing everything possible while striving for perfection. The devolution of our quality of life, however, has made us weaker, with constant bombardment by toxins, noise, and irritated people that can make our lives miserable.

People with stressful family lives often have the genetics for thyroid abnormality (family history of diabetes, rheumatoid arthritis, colitis, migraine, early graying of hair, left-handedness, other autoimmune conditions).

We suggest that you find ways to minimize the chores—and people—
that bring you down and make you feel worse.

Consider the areas in your life where you feel drained. Make a pie
chart of your life and assign percentages to the various pieces. If too much
of your energy is going toward chores that drain you, do not just wonder
why you are feeling drained, do something about it!

Work with that pie chart, until you can get the draining chores and
people sliced down to a minimum. You may not be able to do much about
the tasks you are required to perform at work, but what about those people you hang out with? Do they energize your life, or do they suck up
your joy?

Energy Drainers

As odd as this may sound, energy vampires are all around us. There are
people who are not necessarily bad (though some are), but who have learned
to get what they want in life through manipulation. Some know they are
doing it, while others may not be aware.

It may seem unusual as a suggestion, but we urge you to clean out the
energy drainers in your life. If there are people who take more than they
give and seem to be using you, you can learn to move on.

- Those that suck up your life force must be handled—and soon!
- If they are your children, let them know what you will and will not
  tolerate from them.
- If it is a partner, elucidate clearly your concerns and requests.
- Be honest in your sharing; keep hearts open.
- Make sure that the other person understands your needs fully.

You cannot fix everyone around you, but you can fix yourself.

Being clear about what is acceptable in your presence can help those
around you to act more favorably.

Set limits with caring. Do whatever is possible in your life to
inspire others to make a difference. Then your life has greater purpose,
your family dysfunction is being healed, and you can relax knowing you
have done your best.

What's at Stake?

What we have seen in our medical office is that people want desperately to feel well, to have the energy to do good work, and to enjoy their lives. Often they are "forwarded" from one practitioner to another, yet seldom evaluated carefully enough to uncover the real underlying problem.

Careful, early diagnosis can save health consumers precious time, enabling them to live a more positive and fruitful life. Careful, early evaluation can save employers vast amounts of money in employee sick time and can boost morale. Caring for ourselves can inspire others.

> **Becoming edgy in midlife can be a genetically related thyroid imbalance.**

How Common Is Anxiety?

- A National Institute of Mental Health survey suggested that **10% of the adult population has suffered from some anxiety disorder** in the preceding 6 months. (Kessler)
- It is estimated that **27% of adults have suffered from an anxiety disorder during their lifetime**. That means that at any one time, nearly 15 million Americans are suffering from an anxiety disorder.

Clearly this is an area of crucial importance.

- Studies have shown that **thyroid issues are very common in highly anxious patients** and their family members. (Lindermann)
- Also, it is well known that anxiety is a common symptom in thyroid patients. Clinicians see it over and over, most commonly in people with high thyroid, but also in those with low thyroid.

The Larger View

Here is how experts categorize edginess:

- Generalized anxiety
- Panic disorder

- Phobia
- Obsessive-compulsive disorder
- Post-traumatic stress disorder

Each of these disorders, according to psychologists, has its own stages of development and its own related causes and triggers. They are surprisingly common. Perhaps some of these terms need to be defined.

- **Anxiety:** A state in which a person has a sense of excessive worry, with a nonspecific or unknown source.
- **Compulsion:** Repetitive behavior or actions, the goal of which is to reduce the distress of anxiety.
- **Fear:** A strong sense of dread, focused on a specific object or event.
- **Generalized anxiety disorder:** Psychiatric illness characterized by excessive anxiety or dread for a significant part of the time.
- **Obsession:** Recurrent thought, experienced as inappropriate or intrusive, causing significant distress or discomfort.
- **Panic disorder:** Psychiatric illness that involves discrete episodes of intense, terrible anxiety, accompanied by extremely disconcerting physical symptoms. These episodes are called *panic attacks*.
- **Phobia:** Persistent, almost overwhelming fear of a specific object.

The Stages of Anxiety

Anxiety is a part of daily life for many of us. The large continuum of severity in any of anxiety's categories can include everything from mild distress to severe panic.

According to a leading psychiatric nursing textbook by Frisch and Frisch, these are the Stages of Anxiety:

- **Stage One: Mild Anxiety.** Tension of day-to-day living.

    Example: You miss the bus and will be late.
- **Stage Two: Moderate Anxiety.** Focus is on an immediate concern, narrowed focus, with some inattention to the larger world around you.

    Example: You are about to take an exam on which you are

feeling pressured to do very well. Acceptance into a certain program rests on these results.

- **Stage Three: Severe Anxiety.** Total focus is on very specific details of the upsetting situation. Perception is greatly reduced.

  Example: You witness a car accident.

- **Stage Four: Panic.** A sense of terror, disorganization, loss of control.

  Example: You experience a major earthquake, then feel "unglued."

Variations of Anxiety

People from different walks of life experience anxiety quite differently because of personal, situational, cultural, or societal factors. Men and women differ remarkably in the ways they express anxiety symptoms, largely based on accepted norms of "masculine" and "feminine" behavior.

People who are anxious view themselves as weak or childish, largely due to traditional societal expectations in the Western world. Men in particular may view anxiety, in themselves or other men, as a sign of diminished masculinity or personal weakness, or perhaps a way of avoiding responsibility.

> As a result, men—more than women—exhibit their anxiety as aggression, anger, or irritability.

Some anxious people are talkative, fearful, sarcastic, or demanding. Others are silent and apathetic when anxious. Frequently, anxiety has physical symptoms. Mild versions of physical complaints can include loss of appetite, dry mouth, and fatigue. More severe forms might involve sweating, shakiness, chest pains, rapid heartbeat, hyperventilation, and vomiting.

We can have a wide range of severity in symptoms. Highly anxious people can have the full range of many of these symptoms, or simply exhibit only one. Sometimes there are no physical symptoms, just a vague sense of fear, dread, apprehension, intolerance, frustration, or overreaction to even mild events.

In addition to these symptoms, there are **telltale behaviors**:

- Compulsions
- Preoccupations

- Repetitive actions (such as nail biting, nervous plucking of hairs, or continually locking windows and doors)

Anxiety symptoms can be highly distressing to one person, yet only mildly distressing to another. The experience of stress is not the same from one person to another.

One highly distressed person might be suffering a great deal but will hide it. In these people, we may be surprised when something drastic happens, but we could better have anticipated it had we paid attention to their small behaviors. Another might discuss his or her distress in colorful detail and not seem at all troubled. People have often developed coping mechanisms to help them get through anxious times. Many do not like when their anxiety shows.

Control Patterns

Many anxious people try to manage their discomfort with anxiety-controlling behaviors:

- Overeating
- Excessive TV watching
- Heavy use of substances like alcohol or marijuana
- Procrastination
- Hoarding

These and other activities are what co-counselors call "control patterns," habits people develop to keep from feeling their feelings. They are frequently used to relieve discomfort from anxiety. They do this by producing an alternative mental state, such as "zoning out" with alcohol, or with apathy and procrastination.

For some people, apathy and procrastination are much less distressing than anxiety, while others cannot even begin to tolerate themselves as apathetic and procrastinating.

Many people continue to use these control patterns, regardless of the long-term negative effects on themselves or others. Often, the long-term result of using anxiety-relieving behaviors is that they eventually contribute to further anxiety states. This additional distress affects not just the person using these behaviors but also all those around him or her.

Because anxiety is such a common human experience, it has long been of interest to psychologists and physicians. These practitioners know that it can ultimately be so severe that it makes people feel as if their lives are not worth living. It is heartening to realize that this whole picture can often be changed for the better by simply improving thyroid balance.

The Age of Anxiety

Given everything we are facing on a global scale, some say we live in the Age of Anxiety. Indeed, it is difficult to imagine how people can live with enhanced awareness of the challenges in our world and *not* have anxiety as a part of their lives. Many psychologists agree that this kind of anxiety might easily become debilitating.

Some disagree, feeling that mild anxiety can be channeled and made useful. For example, it can help to properly negotiate a dangerous situation. This may have been true in other times, but today the fears that plague us are enormous. They range from something immediate and potentially imminent, like identity theft, to the looming specter of global warming, with floods and relocation of populations. Today's issues are such huge problems that it is hard to focus on them in a sensible way and not live with anxiety.

Mild anxiety is often considered an acceptable part of social function in industrialized cultures, but extreme anxiety has been shown to severely limit human potential.

Study after study documents severe impairment in quality of life when a person suffers from significant anxiety, which includes many of us.

The Side Effects of Edgy Living

For most people, being edgy is an unpleasant state of physical and psychological arousal that interferes with effective social function. It also affects their ability to interact with others, to develop healthy relationships, and to enjoy success at work.

Our experience with anxiety ranges from mild and occasional, to severe anxiety as a continual behavior pattern. Some people just seem to be high strung. Their anxiety manifests as a predictable severe response to any stress.

Mild anxiety is simply part of regular life for many people. For some it can be a positive motivating force. For others, however, and especially when severe or chronic, anxiety can become medically risky and debilitating.

People differ widely in how they experience and communicate anxiety. These differences reflect personal variations in learned behavior. They also reflect personal variations in hormone levels and function.

Edginess in Daily Life

If you were raised in an unstable family environment, with serious emotional outbursts, we specifically reach out to you. We hope the science and stories encourage you to consider a thyroid mental tune-up. The mind may need tuning at various times, just as surely as a car, and many aspects of our lives require ongoing maintenance.

If your sense of security, peace of mind, or overall well-being has been undermined; if you are ready to restore your brain to a greater level

Karilee's Corner

Karilee worked for many years in psychiatric facilities. Some of these units were a part of a hospital, while others were independent. Some were excellent, providing superior care, while others were amazingly lucrative for the owners, at surprisingly poor advantage to the client.

One of her strongest memories was of a girl name Earline, who had stick-straight hair, Coke-bottle glasses, and obvious nervous twitches and tics, the latter made even worse by her psychiatric medications. Her family brought her regularly to a day treatment program that provided a therapeutic environment for those with mental/emotional challenges.

One morning in group therapy session, Karilee suggested that for the next day, each client should bring in a family photograph.

Out of all the family pictures presented by clients, Earline's photo took her breath away.

There was her mother, neat and prim, arms leaning over her

of mental health, and **if you have the mental challenge of excess worry or nervousness and have not been** *carefully* **checked for thyroid imbalance, please do so.** Refer to Chapter 3 and request the full panel of blood tests and other diagnostic maneuvers. Finding and treating your thyroid issue can often free you from the grip of anxiety.

If you are currently being treated for low or high thyroid with some success, but are still bothered by strong anger or fear, consider that your thyroid correction could benefit from further improvement. You might try some of the ideas in our treatment section later in this chapter.

> **Pay close attention to** *any* **remaining mental symptoms, no matter how slight, that may linger after thyroid's physical challenges are relieved.**

Many people seek out doctors to help them with the physical symptoms of thyroid problems. Often, with medication, they feel better and get relief from those symptoms. They may, however, later notice that the mental realm could benefit from further fine-tuning with even better thyroid care.

---

fashionably dressed husband, encircled by three other children, all doll-like. Suddenly, almost silently, a figure called from the other side of the frame.

It was a girl, curved over, hair dangling, with a back so rounded that it appeared exhausted, bent from carrying the weight of her life. This girl, Earline, stood all alone, apart, away from the others. Due to her extreme edginess, she lived outside the family circle and had learned to endure.

We learned years later that Earline had been diagnosed with hypothyroidism and that with thyroid care, both she and her family were now doing much better. Wherever you are now, Earline, in this beautiful and challenging Earth realm, we envision you moving with a new grace and ease that you have earned.

We see you now as comfortable in your body, accepting of your life at this time. We visualize you without the tragic hormonal anxiety that at first seemed to paralyze your world, keeping you locked inside yourself. Mostly, we see you surrounded by love.

A Look at the Science

For some people, no amount of documentation is sufficient. For others, none is necessary. Those who appreciate the beauty of science might enjoy the research and practice findings here. To those less interested, we invite you to simply move on to the next section.

High Thyroid Edginess

Most seasoned practitioners have long been aware of a considerable connection between anxiety and thyroid disorders. From the very first description of high thyroid, 180 years ago, anxiety symptoms were viewed as a part of this condition.

The author of that original article from 1835 was the renowned physician Dr. Robert James Graves, for whom Graves' disease (high thyroid) was named. Ever since these early descriptions of hyperthyroidism, symptoms prominently featured were agitation, anxiety, restlessness, and nervousness. (Graves)

Practicing physicians have continued to note a strong correlation between anxiety and high thyroid situations. Correlations have been variously recorded in medical journals, lectures, and textbooks. (Wartofsky)

Not all anxiety is caused by thyroid imbalance, but plenty of it is, enough to make us anxious about the situation. (Katerndahl)

Across the country, and perhaps around the world, endocrinology clinics offer opportunity for observation of rampant anxiety disorders in patients with hyperthyroidism, and occasionally hypothyroidism. In some of these patients, the anxiety resolves completely with thyroid treatment. (Cathol)

Many other clinicians have reported this co-occurrence of **panic attacks in patients with hyperthyroidism or hypothyroidism**. Conversely, it is also commonly reported by psychiatrists that many of their patients with panic disorder have hyper- or hypothyroidism causing their problem. (Stein)

Ever since the 1980s, specialists have considered it medically prudent to carefully **check for thyroid dysfunction in**

patients with anxiety disorders or panic attacks. Primary care practitioners, however, do not always check carefully enough for this thyroid cause.

- An **excess of thyroid hormone** will cause rapid heartbeat, tightness of muscles, insomnia, as well as a sense of extreme stress and anxiety. Too much thyroid hormone throttles the system into extra-fast metabolism, with hyperarousal of mental state. (Landsberg)

- The actual **hyperarousal neurotransmitter** acting in the brains of certain high and low thyroid people might be noradrenaline, rather than the adrenaline secreted from the adrenal medulla. It is well known that in severe hypothyroidism, the sympathetic nervous system tends to be overly active. (Landsberg)

- Sometimes in nervousness and anxiety, the **distinction between hyper- and hypothyroid is a source of confusion.** Both kinds of patients can have palpitations and emotional upsets at the slightest provocation. (Iranmanish)

The Low Thyroid–Anxiety Connection

It is a bit more challenging to see how low thyroid could cause the high arousal of anxiety, but it does. Low metabolism can have this effect because of the body's attempt to compensate.

> *Hypo*thyroidism causes anxiety problems due to abnormal noradrenaline and serotonin levels in specific areas of the brain, as well as adrenal gland compensation.

- According to many recent studies, a significant percentage of **low thyroid patients present themselves as nervous and apprehensive.** (de Groot)

- When one energy hormone, such as thyroid, is low, the **compensatory mechanism** is to release more of another energy hormone.

This is often cortisol, adrenaline, or both. These latter two come from the adrenal gland, trying to compensate for a sluggish thyroid. (Ungar)

- The result is that you may **have more energy to get through your day, but it comes at the price of greater edginess**, a result of extra amounts of adrenal hormones. This effect of low thyroid is often confused with high thyroid. (Goldberg)

- Thyroid hormone, as a source of energy for the body, is preferred over adrenaline as a source of energy. Adrenaline is best utilized for fight-or-flight situations.

- When adrenaline is utilized for daily energy due to lowered thyroid hormone, the person experiences its side effects, which can be anxiety and nervousness. (Kamilaris)

The Chemistry of Fear

What is really going on in the brains and minds of people with thyroid imbalances?

Both the *cerebral cortex* (our under-the-hat computer) and the upper brain stem *limbic system* (the seat of emotions) are involved in our fear response and in the emotions related to it.

When anxious people are observed during a sophisticated scanning procedure (PET scan), the actual amount of blood flow to specific areas of the brain is shown. When anxiety occurs, the PET scan shows an increase in blood flow to the limbic system and specific areas of the cerebral cortex.

What could be happening in these areas during heightened blood flow? Certain chemicals are understood by experts to be the main mood regulators, especially serotonin, which is considered a key player in mood symptoms and mood disorders. Research studies have shown that there are specific serotonin subgroups, and subtypes of those subgroups, which have been identified and correlated with specific changes in mood.

Anxiety is correlated to changes in level, effectiveness, or receptor sensitivity of three key neurotransmitters: norepinephrine, serotonin, and GABA.

The search for more precise biochemical explanations of anxiety is ongoing.

- One result of some of this investigation is that the newer **serotonin reuptake inhibitor** (SSRI) antidepressants have been found helpful for relieving some anxieties.
- Specific anxiety-relieving medications also include **benzodiazepines,** the first one being Valium. This category now includes a long list of tranquilizer drugs.
- Also helpful for anxiety is the group of drugs known as **beta-blockers.** These are generally older, safer, and well-tested drugs initially developed as a way of lowering high blood pressure but **later found to work in relieving anxiety symptoms from an excessively aroused sympathetic nervous system.** These symptoms include rapid heart rate, sweating, and involuntary muscle contractions (tremors or shaking), all symptoms of the *sympathetic* portion of the *autonomic nervous system.* Recall that the autonomic nervous system is divided into two main parts:
  - **Parasympathetic** nervous system, which slows the body and heart down
  - **Sympathetic** nervous system, which is related to arousal, speeding things up, and increasing the intensity

The medicines thus far mentioned do not have a direct mood effect per se, but instead seem to either relax the body (beta-blockers) or tone down the brain (tranquilizers). **Beta-blockers block some of the sympathetic nervous system transmissions.** Like benzodiazepines, they relieve anxiety symptoms, without actually treating the underlying condition that actually produced the anxiety in the first place.

One particular drug from a different category, specifically **marketed for anxiety,** is called BuSpar. As we will see later in the chapter, thyroid hormone might sometimes be an even better antianxiety medication than this, or any of the above.

There is **often a high prevalence of thyroid illness in the family history of the affected "anxious" person,** although blood tests do not always reflect it. With more accurate testing, including thyroid antibodies and possible TRH testing, a closer clinical concurrence may ultimately be revealed. (As mentioned in Chapter 3, TRH testing is expensive but very accurate and often used in research.)

Brain researchers studying anxiety have found signs of **noradrenaline hyperfunction**, frequently improved with beta-blocking drugs. High thyroid is also associated with **increased alpha-adrenaline receptor binding** and **altered noradrenaline turnover**. (Atterwill)

An interesting suggestion about the link between thyroid and noradrenaline function is derived from evidence that **noradrenaline serves as a neurotransmitter, regulating immune response**. Changes in noradrenaline transmission clearly alter the immune function, perhaps by a direct effect on the immune cell receptors, or by modulating levels of lymphokines. (Felten)

This immune response may explain why people have bouts of autoimmune thyroid disease when severely stressed. It also explains why, for so many years, practicing clinical physicians have observed onset or worsening of thyroid problems after times of anxiety, nervousness, and stress.

The difficulty in lab diagnosis of abnormal thyroid in anxiety patients might be due to one crucial fact:

> Levels of thyroid hormone in a blood draw provide only a crude relationship to what is actually occurring inside any particular organ.

At a given target tissue, such as the brain, there may be either hyper- or hypothyroidism, with normal levels of circulating thyroid hormone in the bloodstream. This means that thyroid blood tests are *not* gospel.

Measuring the level of antibodies gives us another correlation to a thyroid cause for edginess. It has been argued that the presence of thyroid antibodies does not in itself prove impairment of thyroid function. Many studies, however, have shown that up to 70% of patients with symptomless autoimmune thyroiditis (showing normal T3, T4, and TSH levels) will have evidence of decreased thyroid reserve. (DeBoel)

The Biology of Mood

Irritability is such a commonly seen symptom of both hyper- and hypothyroidism that some authors have suggested considering thyroid imbalance as the best naturally occurring model of the biology of mood. (Fundaro)

- One study examined the course and severity of thyroid antibodies over time in anxiety-disordered people. It was found that **anxiety rises and falls with the rise and fall of thyroid antibodies**.

- Further studies by the same author used TRH testing in addition to thyroid antibody testing. The results led the authors to propose greater use of TRH testing in psychiatry in general. Early on, it was the study authors' hope that the development of the ultra-sensitive TSH testing would ultimately be as useful as the more expensive TRH test, but this has not proven to be the case.

- Other researchers have conducted studies on the **favorable use of T3 thyroid hormone in patients with panic disorder** who were poorly responsive to standard psychiatric medications. This research is similar to that showing **a good T3 thyroid hormone response in depressed patients** who were not helped enough by regular antidepressant medicines.

- One study found that 27% of male veterans diagnosed with post-traumatic stress disorder (PTSD) had abnormal thyroid testing. (Kosten)

- Another intriguing piece of research found that **patients with panic disorder** who were being **successfully treated with amitriptyline** (Elavil) had significant changes in the TSH response to TRH, hence they were thyroid unbalanced. (Stein)

- Patients with **panic disorder** have been found to exhibit a **remission** of symptoms **during pregnancy**. (George) Another study observed the **worsening** or new onset of panic attack in **postpartum** women. (Metz) This pattern of remission during pregnancy and worsening afterward is consistent with the typical course of thyroiditis. This condition can cause either high or low thyroid, but it is mild, or mostly gone, during pregnancy. It suddenly reappears or becomes worse in the postpartum period.

This striking correlation in timing **suggests a clear link between panic attacks and thyroid problems**, regardless of what the blood tests show.

What Can We Learn?

Anxiety disorders can be triggered or worsened by thyroid disorders.

It is highly unfortunate that thyroid imbalance so frequently remains undiagnosed. Treating the thyroid disorder often resolves much or all of the edginess.

The result is that *far too many people* are experiencing ongoing anxiety and are not receiving appropriate treatment. In light of all this information, it is quite clear that **better diagnosis and treatment of thyroid imbalance should be a bigger part of the treatment of anxiety issues.**

Our Treatment Recommendations
Over-the-Counter Remedies for Low Thyroid

Considering the many types of natural thyroid boosters, the one with the best track record for the Edgy person is **porcine thyroid glandular**. This is sold at most health food and vitamin stores as bottles of tablets, each containing from 50 to 150 mg of thyroid tissue. This main ingredient is often combined with other glandulars, vitamins, minerals, or amino acids.

- It is our recommendation that you **choose the highest quality version** of this complex product that you can find and afford. Frequently, this involves ordering direct from a top nutraceutical company. Patients at our clinic have been most satisfied with the preparation called **T-150** from Xymogen (see page 279).
- Another version that has been highly successful is **Thytrophin** by Standard Process. Some people find that this, or the T-150, works for them *as well as, or better than, prescription* thyroid medicine. Others find they can take less prescribed medicine by virtue of also taking thyroid glandular.

Start with one pill once a day in the morning. This is all that some people will ever need. Many, however, find this starting dose too light for ongoing treatment. Instead, they will increase by one additional pill daily, every 2 weeks. Usually a sufficient effect is noticed at three or four pills per day, taken all at once in the morning, well before breakfast.

If you have slowly tapered up to four pills daily without apparent effect, you may need to boost your over-the-counter medicine with some nutritional co-factors. Thyroid frequently works best with adequate selenium, magnesium, zinc, carnosic acid (usually from rosemary extract), and vitamin D.

- Multiple co-factors like these are conveniently combined at their effective doses in products such as **MedCaps T3** by Xymogen, and **Thyrosol** by Metagenics. Two or three pills daily of either of these thyroid boosters is an excellent complement to your glandular program.

Sometimes the co-factor most needed for optimal effect from the thyroid glandular is *adrenal cortex support.* Irritable and nervous thyroid sufferers are commonly low in adrenal cortex hormones. This situation can often be best remedied with a mix of vitamins and herbal medicines, targeted for the care and feeding of adrenal function.

- The vitamins of choice for this purpose are **high doses of B_5 with a small amount of B_6.** The best herbals proven to be helpful in this case are the **adaptogenic herbs**, including ginseng, rhodiola, cordyceps, bacopa, and a few others. Once again, for convenience and highest quality, we recommend **Corticare B** and **Adrenal Essence** from Xymogen, or **Cortico-B_5B_6** and **Adreset** by Metagenics.

Over-the-Counter Remedies for High Thyroid

Several standard supplements that are routinely utilized for other purposes can, at higher doses, serve to lower thyroid hormone production. Including one or more of these in your program to lower a *hyper*thyroid situation can serve you optimally.

- The first item to consider is the amino acid **L-carnitine**. At doses above 3 grams per day, it begins to have antithyroid effects. This could be a problem for a low thyroid person, but can be very helpful for high thyroid people. It comes as a 500-mg pill, so you start with two pills three times per day. If more thyroid-lowering effect is needed after several weeks at this dose, you can increase to three pills three times daily.
- Of similar antithyroid effect is the bioflavonoid **quercetin**. This also is often sold as a 500-mg pill; doses above 3 grams can lower thyroid hormone production. Like carnitine, doses below this level rarely have this side effect. The procedure for utilizing quercetin is the same as for carnitine.

- Another item that will lower thyroid function is **lipoic acid**. Even though it is not strongly acidic, it is an exceptionally good antioxidant. Unlike some other antioxidants, however, above 500 mg per day, it can begin to lower thyroid hormone production as a side effect. For people who want to utilize this side effect to their advantage, a dose of 600 to 800 mg per day will be a very useful addition to their program.

- Still another common and generally benign item is **soy**. More than 50 mg per day of soy isoflavones, however, can lower thyroid hormone production. This seems to be especially true for people who are taking thyroid medicine. For that reason, we have not recommended much soy for those with low thyroid. However, for those with high thyroid, soy can be a fine addition. Taking 75 to 100 mg per day of soy isoflavones will help reduce high thyroid hormone levels.

Prescription Treatment of Low Thyroid

Of all the many different thyroid medicines, the best treatment for an Edgy person who has thyroid imbalance is to start with **levothyroxine**. This is the standard T4 thyroid hormone available as brand names Synthroid, Levoxyl, Levothroid, and Unithroid. Good generic alternatives to the brand name products come from drug manufacturers like Sandoz, Lannett, and Mylan.

Straight levothyroxine is the best choice in anxiety or irritability. Of all the off-the-shelf thyroid medicines, it is the *least likely to create further edginess* by irritating the adrenal system. T3 is needed ultimately, but in these anxiety situations, it is best derived from the intracellular conversion of T4 to T3 within the body.

In our clinic we have found that many people with anxiety caused by high or low thyroid also have adrenal cortex insufficiency. This problem of the adrenal cortex results in episodes of excessive output of adrenal medulla hormones like adrenaline, noradrenaline, and dopamine. The last thing Edgy people need is to have worse adrenal symptoms due to harsh thyroid treatment.

Thyroxine is best for this situation because it is so slow acting, and slow to accumulate in the body. This gives the system time to adapt to the increasing levels of thyroid hormone resulting from treatment. If the treatment were, for instance, the fast-acting T3 thyroid hormone (brand Cytomel, or generic liothyronine) or the moderately fast-acting Armour-type desiccated thyroid, then the possibility for unmasking and worsening adrenal insufficiency would be greater.

The experience of unmasking adrenal insufficiency can be quite uncomfortable, with rapid heart rate, tremor, sweating, headache—a generalized hyped-up feeling that is the total opposite of the sought-after effect. For this reason, many practitioners like to check adrenal function before giving thyroid hormone. This is especially appropriate for anxiety-prone people, who may already have disrupted adrenal gland function.

An accurate way to check adrenal status is to do the standard saliva test. This consists of giving a sample of saliva for testing of cortisol and DHEA at four different times in 1 day. Home test kits are easily available for this purpose, with results being more accurate than standard morning and/or afternoon blood tests. You can self-order your own adrenal function test by going to www.CanaryClub.org.

If your adrenal test is fine, or if you choose to start thyroid medicine without adrenal testing, the prudent method of taking the medicine is to **start low and go slow.** Ask your practitioner to start you off with a very small amount of thyroxine, say 25 mcg. This is the smallest strength pill available off the shelf. Stay with one pill once a day in the morning for a week, then increase to two pills a day in the morning. Remain at this plateau for several weeks.

If low thyroid was causing your edginess and irritability, then this level of thyroid hormone should result in noticeable improvement after a few weeks. Some people notice the improvement much sooner than that, but not everyone. Stay at this dose for several weeks and see if you feel better as time goes on. Thyroxine is so slow to accumulate that it can be 6 to 8 weeks before the full effect of this dose is reached.

At the end of this period, **if you are not feeling better**, then increase to 75 mcg a day for another 6 to 8 weeks. If still no better, go up to 100 mcg a day, and see how this feels after another 6 weeks. If still no better at all, then it is unlikely that thyroxine is an optimal thyroid medicine for you.

If, on the other hand, you do feel improved, but the improvement at smaller doses (like 50 mcg) was short-lived, then you can try more. If that improvement lasted longer and felt better, but later faded, then you could increase even further.

The stepwise increase of 25 mcg at a time is called slow upward titration. We consider this the proper way for a person with excess anxiety to receive levothyroxine.

If 100 mcg reacted similarly by giving some definite, but only temporary, relief from the edginess, then you might well increase the thyroxine dose further. Occasionally, people need up to 1 mcg of thyroxine per pound of body weight (so if you weigh 150 pounds, you would need 150 mcg). Most people do well with less than that maximum dose.

Find the dose at which *your* body feels best.

When it comes to thyroid medicine, more is not better. What is better is to *find just the right amount* that is optimal for your system.

If anywhere on this upward taper you start to feel more anxious and hyped up, there are two options to consider:

1. It could be that you are taking more thyroxine than your body needs (becoming slightly hyperthyroid).
2. You could be unmasking adrenal insufficiency. Generally no one becomes truly hyperthyroid on 25, 50, or even 75 mcg of thyroxine.

If you start feeling hyper on these modest doses of thyroxine, you might not be hyperthyroid; you might simply be adrenal insufficient. The addition of adrenal boosters to your thyroid medicine can remedy this situation, leaving you feeling a whole lot better.

Prescription Treatment of High Thyroid

Many of the symptoms experienced by an Edgy person can be caused fully, or in part, by too much thyroid hormone in the system. Standard medical management of this condition involves the use of antithyroid medicines, radioactive iodine (RAI) treatment to ablate the gland, or removal of thyroid gland by surgery.

We will not be discussing these last two options here in detail. Several other fine books are available for this purpose, including *Living Well with Graves' Disease and Hyperthyroidism* by Mary Shomon, and *Graves' Disease: A Practical Guide* by Elaine Moore. The Shomon book contains more of the Shames's recommendations specifically for this condition.

Most people diagnosed with Graves' high thyroid are advised to have surgery or radioactive ablation as a first step. We have "grave" concerns about that advice!

High thyroid is sometimes the early temporary phase of the Hashimoto's low thyroid condition, though this is often overlooked. Be sure that your practitioners have an absolute ironclad antibody diagnosis of Graves' disease before giving you either of the permanent maneuvers.

If the natural remedies listed above are not helpful enough, many people should instead be given the opportunity to first try **antithyroid medicines**, like **PTU** (propylthiouracil) or **Tapazole** (methimazole). These chemicals will slow down the thyroid gland's production of thyroid hormone and bring the system back to normalcy.

Endocrinology doctors most often advise their patients to have the more definitive surgery or radioactive treatment right away, because they feel that the hyperthyroid condition soon returns after the medicine is stopped.

We strongly suggest that you firmly ask your doctor for a trial of PTU or Tapazole as a first step in the ongoing process of getting your thyroid situation under control. You can always do the permanent procedures of either RAI or surgery at a later time, if the antithyroid medicines have not resulted in long-term improvement. You cannot, however, restore a gland that has been irradiated or removed.

Before accepting a diagnosis of Graves' hyperthyroidism, **you need to ask for and *see* abnormally high results** on either or both of the two **Graves' antibody tests**:

- TSI (thyroid-stimulating immunoglobulin)
- TBII (thyrotropin-binding inhibitory immunoglobulin)

If these antibodies do not show that you have actual Graves' disease, you are likely to have a temporary high phase of Hashimoto's thyroiditis.

This will often burn out of the high phase in a matter of weeks and then begin to revert to its standard low thyroid presentation. In this situation, with Hashimoto's temporarily resulting in high thyroid, the treatment is to simply relieve symptoms of shakiness, insomnia, and rapid pulse until this phase resolves. The Hashimoto's situation does not necessarily need extreme measures to block production of thyroid hormone.

Be certain of your actual diagnosis before resorting to drastic permanent measures, like surgery or radioactive treatments, with their own risks and consequences.

Suppose your antibodies are indeed diagnostic of Graves'. It is our basic recommendation for people with this kind of high thyroid to choose one of the two antithyroid medicines, **Tapazole** or **PTU**, as a first step.

> **Tapazole** (methimazole) is best started at a very low dose, perhaps one 5-mg pill per day, unless the high thyroid is severe. If it is severe, doctors will generally start a patient at 10 to 15 mg. Starting at the lower dose of 5 mg per day and working up slowly as needed is our preferable approach. Elevated levels of thyroid hormone can be reduced by Tapazole, but side effects can be harmful to the liver or blood cells, especially at higher doses. A simple blood test can check for these side effects.

> **PTU** (propylthiouracil) is also effective at reducing thyroid hormone production by the thyroid gland. It also has similar side effects and is currently being used less than Tapazole. Starting dose for PTU can be 50 mg. An eventual dose of 100 mg three times a day is common for severe cases. As with Tapazole, it is best to use a small amount when possible.

And that brings us to the benefits of natural over-the-counter products, as discussed above.

Supplementation

We strongly suggest that your best option when it is necessary to use Tapazole or PTU is to **combine that prescription treatment with over-the-counter antithyroid supplements**. The combined effect will allow you to get the same hormone-lowering result with less of the expensive prescription chemical, and with less harmful side effects.

You should stay on the antithyroid medicines for a year or two, as long as they are well tolerated and blood tests are normal. After this time, ask to have your dose gradually tapered down over a couple of months. Then you can be retested for the presence of high thyroid.

Often the high thyroid condition will become resolved and will remain so, especially if you have been combining the prescription medicine with natural recommendations.

Complementary Healing for Your Best Results

By Georjana Shames, LAc

Previously we discussed how the ancient Chinese system of the Five Elements encompasses Fire, Earth, Metal, Water, and Wood. You have seen how the Moody type of thyroid imbalance relates to the Fire element (and Heart Meridian). Now we discuss how the Edgy type of imbalance relates to the Wood element (and Liver Meridian).

The Liver Meridian is responsible for the smooth flow of the emotions in Acupuncture theory; thus it is the most susceptible to stagnation caused by stress.

Irritability, anger, and rage result from Liver Meridian stagnation.

Remember that occasionally feeling an appropriate amount of anger can be a fine thing. It can be the impetus one needs to change an unhealthy situation or to take action about an issue that is bothersome. Anger in excess (such as rage or constant feelings of irritation) can wreak destructive havoc on your life, causing you to live in a state of perpetual stress and mental chaos.

And here's the kicker:

If you are an Edgy type, even when you properly regulate your thyroid, it may still be necessary to rewire your stress response to avoid a life of Liver Meridian stagnation.

In other words, severe rage attacks can often be decreased with proper thyroid care, but the underlying pattern of stagnation within the Liver Meridian needs to be addressed to create a more peaceful life.

Here are some points you can press on your body to assist Liver Meridian:

• Locate the tender spot on the top of the foot between the great toe and the second toe, about half an inch down from the margin of the web. Press this point (called Liver 2) whenever excessive anger starts to arise. This point cools Liver Fire (rage), and the more tender the point feels, the more you need this pressure at that moment. You could press deeply enough that it really catches your attention and stops the cyclical flaring of rage.

- Locate another tender spot directly below Liver 2, about an inch and a half further down the instep, distal to the junction of the metatarsal bones. Press this area (called Liver 3) whenever anxiety and depression arise. This point "courses the Liver energy," meaning it breaks through stagnation and restores the free flow of the emotions, which is especially helpful in long-standing edginess.

Furthermore, there is a *paired point to Liver 3*, which assists it in the function of restoring free flow of the energy within the body.

- Locate the tender area on the back of the hand in the fleshy depression between thumb and forefinger. The spot you are looking for is located at the highest point of the mound of muscle when you press your thumb against the side of your hand. This point (called Large Intestine 4) is paired with Liver 3, and bilaterally they are called "The Four Gates." Open the gates to remove obstruction, thus restoring the smooth flow of energy throughout the body. **Note: Do not press this point if you are pregnant.**

Massage these points to break long-standing patterns of stagnation in the Liver Meridian. Your emotions will be more balanced, and your mood more tolerant.

RECIPES AND REMEDIES

- Actually, one of the most effective food treatments for the Edgy type of imbalance is to **sip on mint tea** throughout the day. Mint is an invigorating, cooling herb that helps remove stagnation in the Liver Meridian.
- A great meal to help calm anxiety or anger would include lots of **cooling green vegetables**, like a romaine and spinach salad topped with mung beans, with slices of watermelon on the side, and a cup of mint tea as the beverage.
- **Avoiding excess stimulants** (like caffeine and sugar) can help as well.

LIFESTYLE LIFTS

Lifestyle approaches for the Edgy type would include **plenty of vigorous exercise**. Whereas the Moody types benefit more from gentle exercise to boost the spirits, the Edgy person needs to blow off steam. An hour per day of vigorous running, rock climbing, dance, team sports like soccer or basketball, and so on, would benefit the Edgy type of person.

- The little things in life do not have to result in you flying into a rage, nor really do the bigger things. Stress comes and goes, anger waxes and wanes, but your relationships with family members, friends, and colleagues are the most important aspects to cultivate for a long and happy life. Learning to manage anger and cope with stress is paramount.

- Acupuncture can be of great help to millions of people who struggle with anger and anxiety, and so can counseling. If, however, you still struggle with edginess, even after your thyroid has been regulated and you have utilized acupuncture, consider adding counseling with a trusted therapist.

Well-trained therapists can offer many techniques and tools to assist you in handling anxiety, panic, or rage. Even a session once every 2 weeks can be incredibly helpful. This is certainly a great option to consider on your journey to full recovery from hormone havoc.

THE BOTTOM LINE

People dealing with anxiety disorders may well have thyroid as a main cause. For this reason, we suggest doing a thorough thyroid workup on any person who appears agitated and anxious.

We also have recommendations to help these people in all aspects of their lives:

- **Learn to live with *less stress***, avoiding as many sources of stress as you can, as often as possible.
- **People differ widely in how they experience and communicate anxiety**, reflecting not only personal variations in learned behavior but also personal variations in hormone levels and function.
- While some folks seem to enjoy dancing on the edge of stress, for others this can cause meltdown. Ideally each person should know

himself or herself and adjust life accordingly to avoid unnecessary stressors.

- **Thyroid issues are very common in highly anxious patients.** Practitioners need to be more suspicious for thyroid problems with anxious patients. Health consumers can also nudge their providers to do better testing to identify any physical cause of anxiety.

- Anxiety often reflects changes in level, effectiveness, or receptor sensitivity for **three key neurotransmitters: norepinephrine, serotonin, and GABA**. These chemicals help the brain to function well and impact the nervous system response, sleep mechanisms, and overall state of relaxation.

- Large numbers of research studies confirm a **strong low and high thyroid connection to anxiety**. Ideally, practitioners would be more alert to this thyroid connection, intervening earlier to avert long-term states of agitation with side effects that are not easy to reverse.

- Not all anxiety is caused by thyroid, but much of it is.

- Anxiety disorders and panic attacks are frequently helped with the addition of thyroid hormone. This can be a simple solution to a very troubling, enduring problem.

- **Anxiety disorders often occur as a result of thyroid imbalance**, especially *general anxiety disorder and panic disorder*. Less common disorders also occur as a result of thyroid imbalance, including social phobias, specific phobias, obsessive-compulsive disorder (OCD), and post-traumatic stress disorder (PTSD).

RECOMMENDED ACTION PLAN

- For over-the-counter treatment of an Edgy mind-type, start with two pills daily of a high-quality balanced **thyroid glandular** (such as T-150 from Xymogen).

- After a week, add two pills daily of evidence-based **thyroid-boosting nutrients** (such as MedCaps T3 by Xymogen).

- If these are not fully helpful, add a **trial of prescription levothyroxine**, the T4 thyroid hormone, from a qualified practitioner.

- Know that some companies, like Lannett or Sandoz, make good generic levothyroxine that is as good as the more expensive brand names.

- For *low* thyroid, the medicine of choice is **levothyroxine**.

- For *high* thyroid, **be certain of your actual diagnosis** before resorting to drastic permanent measures, like surgery or radioactive treatments, each with their own risks and consequences. Consider the drugs **Tapazole** or **PTU** as a first step.
- Add recommended natural over-the-counter products to complement the prescription treatment.
- When considering medications and products, **find the dose at which *your* body feels best**.
- **Remember:** Before accepting a diagnosis of Graves' hyperthyroidism, **ask for and see abnormally high results** on either or both of the two **Graves' antibody tests**:

  —TSI (thyroid-stimulating immunoglobulin)

  —TBII (thyrotropin-binding inhibitory immunoglobulin)

6

The FOGGY Mind-Type
Improve Attention Deficit, Memory Loss, and Dementia

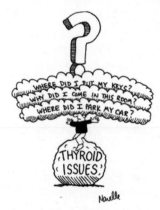

Nora's Story

After several routine years in senior housing, Nora's mind suddenly snapped. She became so fidgety and flighty that the medical center at the facility was increasingly unable to contain her.

She had not responded to the usual medications; her attention span was rapidly growing shorter. She could focus on eating for only a few moments, then insisted she needed to write a letter. All this from a woman who lived to eat in her earlier years!

Grabbing pen and paper, she would write only a few words, then she next switched to reviewing the latest entries in her checkbook. After only

(continued)

a moment of focus, the checkbook was put down because of the sudden need to make a phone call. On it went, as Nora flitted from one thing to another, like an anxiously driven honeybee in a field of blooming flowers.

This new behavior was strikingly different from her previous mild-mannered, prim and proper demeanor. She had for 78 previous years led a calm, well-organized life. Each year, her methodically planned birthday card file was the envy of friends and relatives.

She had been the matriarch, a competent manager of the purse strings. Arguably, she had been the prime force holding a very large family together.

Now, however, she was completely unable to place a stamp on an envelope. What's worse, the medical practitioners were now considering transferring her out of the senior housing complex and into a psychiatric hospital. This was where Tillie stepped in.

Tillie was Nora's daughter, who had recently been surfing thyroid sites on the Internet. Diagnosed with low thyroid 2 years before, at age 56, Tillie had wondered whether her mom's sudden mental change might be thyroid related.

She arm-twisted the facility's doctor to order a complete thyroid panel, despite Nora's normal TSH thyroid screening test. Sure enough, the panel's Free T3 hormone level came back abnormally elevated. Nora was mildly *hyper*thyroid.

This diagnosis had previously been missed, because in early hyperthyroidism, T3 commonly becomes abnormal sooner than TSH. Once the thyroid imbalance had been treated, and the hormone level returned to normal, Nora's mind returned. She was her old self once again.

She had not suffered a nervous breakdown or temporal lobe stroke. Neither did she have attention deficit disorder, nor the rapid onset of Alzheimer's.

Nora simply had thyroid imbalance, as does one in every four postmenopausal women (an eye-opening statistic from the January 2001 *Journal of Epidemiology*). In her particular case, the major resulting thyroid symptom was tremendous loss of focus. Many people with thyroid imbalance have different symptoms.

She did not require expensive psychotropic medicine, and she was certainly not a candidate for the psychiatric hospital. She was, however, headed in that direction, which at her age could have sent her into a permanent downward spiral, like the dean's mother in Chapter 1.

Instead, Tillie had encouraged Nora's doctor to uncover the true diagnosis. With thyroid treatment Nora soon returned to her old self.

What's at Stake?

Focus is a vexing *issue* for many.

Memory difficulties and *outright dementia* **are now in epidemic proportion.** Alzheimer's disease, for example, now affects one out of every eight people over age 65, and almost half of those over age 85. (Riven)

This chapter presents the strong thyroid connections to each of these cognitive mental challenges. We will first look at the hormonal basis for concentration and attention deficits, then move to a discussion of everyday memory loss, finally ending with a discussion of actual dementia.

Attention Deficit Disorder

Most attention deficit situations are not generally as serious or as acute as in Nora's case. In many of those affected, the symptoms can be a mild decrease in one of the so-called executive functions, properties of the mammalian brain that allow certain warm-blooded animals to prioritize, plan, and concentrate awareness on separate related tasks for the appropriate length of time. Attention deficit is both a symptom and a cause of the loss of executive function in our society, in the sense that excess demands being put upon us are making it harder and harder for us to function and focus well.

As it worsens, attention deficit can progress to confusion, diminished capabilities, and eventually even mental breakdown. People in this state can pose a serious health risk to themselves and to others. Beyond the mild stage, the condition is called attention deficit disorder, or simply ADD. With excessive motor component, it becomes attention-deficit/hyperactivity disorder, or ADHD.

ADD often worsens as we age and frequently continues to go unrecognized, largely because *mild thyroid imbalance is regularly confused with normal aging.* There is nothing "normal" about the way many Americans are aging in today's modern world!

According to Ridha Arem, MD, editor of the journal *Thyroid* and a respected endocrinologist and endocrinology professor, nearly 45% (almost half!) of older people have some degree of thyroid gland inflammation, characteristic of Hashimoto's thyroiditis. Dr. Arem further suggests that minor thyroid imbalances often produce greater disturbances in the elderly population than in younger people. (Arem)

Either of these mental conditions is associated with significantly increased coexisting psychological issues. In addition, the likelihood of eventually having ADD or ADHD is greater if someone else in your family previously had it.

In past years, Ritalin was the drug of choice for ADHD in children. Today, many treated with Ritalin as children now have troublesome ADD as adults.

Amazingly, a definite percentage of today's attention deficit problem could be reversed with the simple addition of thyroid hormone.

More people need to become aware of the pervasive and dramatic thyroid aspect of attention and memory.

Dr. Arem confirms his support of studies showing that an imbalance of thyroid hormone in the brain can be responsible for attention-deficit/hyperactivity disorder. It has also been shown that the presentation of thyroid imbalance in adults is what is currently often described as ADD.

Many doctors believe that only severe thyroid abnormality could cause attention deficit or other cognitive loss. Actually, as in Nora's example, *any* degree of thyroid imbalance can, at times, result in sufficient brain dysfunction to cause attention deficit disorder. Even mild impairment of thyroid function is highly associated with this mental condition.

People with attention deficit disorders are causing undue havoc on themselves and the world at large. Many are involved in auto accidents or house fires. Others are disruptive at home or at work. They require extra energy from those around them in social situations, including camp, church, picnics, and, most devastatingly for all concerned, school.

Attention-Deficit/ Hyperactivity Disorder

The prevalence of attention deficit in children is increasing, now close to 7% of all children. In this younger population, it commonly appears as attention-deficit/hyperactivity disorder, or ADHD.

ADHD is a "persistent pattern of inattention or hyperactive impulsivity, interfering with social functioning, school activity, and work performance."

In children, the hyperactivity is expressed as:

- Fidgeting or squirming while seated
- Not wanting to remain seated when expected to do so
- Excessive running or climbing at inappropriate times

In adults, this same condition gives us these symptoms:

- Restlessness
- Difficulty engaging in quiet activities
- Difficulty focusing on one task for the time necessary to complete it
- Impatience while waiting; interrupting frequently; intruding on others to the point of causing disturbance
- Impulsive behavior that can result in engaging in potentially dangerous activities, without thinking of possible consequences

We need to consider the possibility of thyroid as a factor in ADHD. We recommend *complete testing first*, then perhaps treating both affected children and affected adults as carefully as possible, to correct the thyroid.

Those affected by ADHD, but not showing positive test results on thyroid panels, could still be candidates for some kind of thyroid intervention. After careful review of

- Symptoms
- Family history
- Related illness
- Physical signs

. . . *then* the likely-to-be-thyroid-compromised individuals could be given a *trial* of small amounts of thyroid hormone.

Commonly, people diagnosed with ADHD as children find in adulthood that being treated with thyroid hormone, even for other symptoms, will markedly improve their attention deficit. This has happened in case after case at our clinic, to the extent that it is one of the improvement expectations we routinely discuss during the first interview.

A great many of our patients have later told us they were gratefully relieved to be given a new lease on life.

- Instead of total frustration with their job, now they are able to get things done and to have good relationships with their co-workers.

- Instead of existing in a home environment filled with piles of unfinished tasks, now they are able to complete their work, living a more comfortable existence.

- Best of all, they have better interpersonal relationships among friends and significant others. These people find that their ability to relate is much more meaningful, and enduring, than ever before.

Everyday Memory Loss

The ADD issues described in Nora's story also reveal the importance of cognition and its relationship to overall brain function.

> *Cognition* **is defined as the process by which a person knows the world and is able to interact with it.**

With advancing age, people often face the **slow onset of multiple cognitive changes**: decreased memory, diminished abstract thinking, loss of judgment, and impaired perception. This slowdown results in a progressive decline of intellectual function and decreased capacity to perform daily activities.

Intellectual capacity does not necessarily have to diminish with advancing age. Many of our well-balanced thyroid patients remain quite sharp, well into their nineties.

Here's how it works. As we grow older, tissues become more susceptible to injury from a variety of external and internal environmental factors. Therefore, in one's golden years, good brain care is more important than previously.

With strong nutrition, sensible exercise, and *optimal thyroid balance*, memory function can continue unabated. The biochemical mechanism for continuing to make new long-term memory is related in part to the proper firing of neurons in the hippocampus. This region of the brain's temporal lobe received its unusual name from its sea horse shape.

If this crucial and delicate region does not have the proper thyroid power, then the laying down of new memory—in any permanent retrievable form—is diminished. Proper thyroid levels are crucial. (Montauk)

Cognitive dysfunction can include a decrease in attention span, as well as sensory misconceptions called illusions. When misconceptions become more severe, they are called hallucinations. (Hayslip)

> **Memory loss is all too often considered an untreatable consequence of old age. This is not true for those who have mental slowness due to an easily treated *thyroid imbalance*.**

There are a variety of well-studied **physical disorders** that can cause alterations in memory, loss of abstract thinking, changes in judgment, and decreased perception. Dementia is a very large category, often wrongly equated with Alzheimer's disease, which is only *one particular type* of dementia.

Dr. Arem, who also wrote *The Thyroid Solution*, describes general mental effects of hypothyroidism as a kind of "brain fog" wherein a person is unable to remember details, names, or events. Sometimes it can be a milder form, but still very annoying, with frequent word retrieval and word recall issues.

Many of our patients describe the difficulty of reading yet not remembering what they have read or not understanding it. At times they try to describe something to another person but are unable to finish the description. Instead they forget what they were talking about in mid-sentence. Some describe the actual inability to concentrate at all.

> **Such difficulties in memory, focus, and concentration are often symptoms of simple over- or underactive thyroid.**

Happily, for millions this can be easily treated with the application of thyroid hormone. Dr. Arem writes, "Hypothyroid patients frequently have some impairment in memory-related ability. The memory deficit and concentration problems often improve with thyroid hormone treatment."

Iodine Concerns

Memory challenges can be seen the world over, especially in places that lack enough iodine for thyroid hormone to be produced by the thyroid gland. In the United States it was found that people who lacked iodine in their diets were more likely to have impaired cognition, providing even more evidence that thyroid is a major player in this situation. (Fierro-Benitez)

Certain practitioners today are giving rather high doses of iodine to thyroid patients in efforts to help them feel better. However, it is far from clear that this is a widely helpful maneuver. Most people in the United States are not now dramatically iodine insufficient, since iodine is added to certain foods. Also, many folks living in the iodine-insufficient regions of the country know now to supplement or use iodized salt.

Based on our office practice, and the extreme sensitivity of many of our thyroid patients, we continue to believe that giving large "loading" doses of iodine is not always wise, for the simple reason that many autoimmune-challenged thyroid patients seem to react terribly to high doses of iodine.

While the iodine-loading test currently popular is performed with a type of iodine that its proponents feel will not harm the patients, we are still not comfortable taking that kind of risk with people who have felt sick for years.

Low-Grade Hypothyroidism

"Don't worry," says the endocrinologist.

How many times have you heard that a person was diagnosed with thyroid—or possibly you were diagnosed—but it was only "mild," it was only "low grade," it was only "borderline low," or it was only a tiny bit in the abnormal range, not requiring treatment now?

Can a person be mildly pregnant?

If you have any test abnormality at all, you may need help.

Recent research has shown that more than 80% of people with low-grade hypothyroidism had impaired memory function. (Haggerty) It should be noted that, in this study of low-grade hypothyroidism, both short-term memory and visual memory were likewise impaired.

Also, keep in mind that this study was conducted on people with low-grade hypothyroidism. You might wonder, as we do, "What amount of memory and focus impairment occurs in people with more severe hypothyroidism?" We eagerly await further research on this crucial topic.

Postpartum Mind Issues

Another life juncture where impaired memory and concentration show up prominently is in **postpartum hypothyroidism**. Many women with postpartum depression actually have a thyroid problem. But of those *known* to have postpartum thyroid, how many show impaired concentration and memory?

Studies show that approximately **70%** of those women who were hypothyroid in the postpartum period were **more careless**, making significantly more mistakes in their care of the baby than women whose thyroid function was normal. Also, **nearly half** of the women with postpartum hypothyroidism had significant **nightmares**, compared with only about 5% of women whose thyroid function was normal.

Elder Issues

A number of physical causes result in progressive decline in intellectual function and in decreased capacity to perform daily activities. Paramount among these is hypothyroidism.

A key aspect of this discussion is the realization that **hypothyroidism is much more common in the elderly population** than in any other group. Trouble with word recall or word retrieval is a well-known symptom of hypothyroidism in all age groups, but especially in the elderly.

Significant forgetfulness is a very common complaint in older adults, as are problems in creating new memories. These challenges can cause decreased ability to perform functions of daily life and are *not normal*—at any age. Commonly, they have a physiological basis that can be improved with treatment.

It is important to differentiate between the **two types of cognitive impairment**—the *reversible* type, for which evaluation and treatment can make things better, and the *irreversible* type, which stays the same or changes only for the worse. Fortunately, Nora had reversible impairment. Now we need to understand what doctors have been (often incorrectly?) calling irreversible cognitive impairment.

Dementia

Multiple cognitive deficits, such as severe memory loss and disturbance in executive function, can combine to become dementia. To qualify for this diagnosis, a person's impairment must be significant enough to cause a clear disturbance in normal life, and it must represent a definite decline from prior levels of function.

- Alzheimer's disease causes over half of the dementia in senior citizens. (Dawes)
- Alzheimer's is now cited as the number one mental health problem among the rapidly aging population.
- *Memory impairment* is part of its presentation, but it also includes *behavioral alterations* such as paranoia, irritability, aggression, anger outbursts, withdrawal, and suspiciousness. (Oppenheim)
- In addition, Alzheimer's includes other behavioral manifestations, such as unintentional fast gait, motor disturbances, and wandering. In later stages, many become bedridden.
- The already large number of people being treated for Alzheimer's (5.3 million) is expected to double by 2030.

The pathology of Alzheimer's involves degenerative brain lesions that are both plaques and neurofibrillary tangles. The plaques and tangles, related to the accumulation of a peptide called beta-amyloid, seem to interfere with the normal repair of nerve cells and with the function of the **crucial neurotransmitter acetylcholine**. This chemical has been identified as an essential component of cognition and memory.

The genetic underpinnings of the condition have been revealed in recent years, showing a hereditary component and revealing that early onset of the disease has different gene and chromosome abnormalities than later onset.

Most people do not receive genetic testing nor do they have biopsies to detect plaques and tangles. **Diagnosis** is made on the basis of **two criteria**:

- Memory impairment
- One or more from the following list:
  - Language disturbance (aphasia)
  - Impaired motor activities (apraxia)
  - Failure to recognize things (agnosia)
  - Disturbance in executive function

These deficits have to be severe enough to impair social and occupational function. They also have to be characterized by gradual onset, with continuing decline.

Most important, the above deficits must not be due to any other systemic condition known to cause dementia, *such as hypothyroidism*. (Frisch)

It is well known that hypothyroidism can cause any or all of the above diminished brain function.

Thyroid imbalance should be *carefully* ruled out before giving a diagnosis of Alzheimer's disease—especially in the absence of positive findings on biopsy, genetic testing, or brain imaging.

The reason for this is dramatic. Alzheimer's disease is a condition where the underlying cause is unknown and long-term successful treatment is practically nonexistent. The medicines commonly used can be acetyl-cholinesterase inhibitors, such as Aricept (donepezil) and Namenda (memantine).

What Is Wrong with These Drugs?

Nothing is wrong with these drugs, **as long as thyroid has been ruled out**. These kinds of drugs generally increase levels of the neurotransmitter acetylcholine, temporarily improving communication between nerve cells. Still, these medications are effective only in very early stages and will merely slow down progress of the illness, not reverse or heal the condition.

Hypothyroidism, on the other hand, is an easily treated reversible condition. It can appear at any age, though it occurs much more frequently in the elderly. Once treated fully, people often can reclaim a great deal of their previous level of function. At the very least, the dementia is much improved.

We wonder how many people are being readily diagnosed with Alzheimer's and immediately put on Aricept, yet are continuing to decline—because thyroid imbalance is a big part of their mental situation.

These people could well be treated with thyroid hormone. Instead of declining, they could improve—rapidly and wholly. The difference in quality of life for these folks, and loved ones, is enormous.

Vascular Causes of Dementia

Another kind of cognitive deficit is vascular dementia, representing almost 20% of all dementias. In one type, hypertension and cardiovascular disease can cause multiple small strokes over a period of time, which gradually result in blocking of arteries. In another type, there is a gradual decreased blood flow, with steady decline in function.

Sometimes these small events are not really noticed, but this can become a more severe problem, with diminished brain blood flow that no one notices, except in terms of cognitive decline. What is interesting about this group of diagnoses is the relation to cardiovascular disease, especially to **cholesterol** problems and **hypertension**, or high blood pressure.

Amazingly, **both cholesterol and high blood pressure conditions frequently improve with the simple treatment of an underlying thyroid problem**. Keep in mind that you must have abnormal thyroid balance for thyroid medicine to actually improve your lipids or your blood pressures.

Thyroid problems are so common in general, and so enormously common in the elderly, that chances of having thyroid imbalance are high. With too little thyroid, your liver is underthrottled, resulting in higher levels of cholesterol, more deposits of plaque in the arteries, and reduced blood flow as a result of these blockages. As for blood pressure, it can increase with either too little or too much thyroid hormone.

Normalizing the thyroid hormone levels often normalizes blood pressure.

Getting thyroid normalized can improve the cholesterol and blood pressure, either of which can improve vascular dementia significantly. Getting thyroid normalized can therefore result in profound *mental* improvements.

Fixing the Autoimmune Situation

Despite all these good reasons for recommending better thyroid care, perhaps the **major reason we suggest thyroid treatment is to improve the autoimmune situation**. Getting older seems to be accompanied by an increase in autoimmunity in general, and by more thyroid autoimmunity in particular.

This increased immune load results in increased growth of *immune complexes*. These are small particles resulting from the clumping of excess antibodies with other materials, implicated in the generalized clogging of microcapillaries in brain tissue. As intricate as this may sound, treating the thyroid situation helps to lower the autoimmune load, improving circulation, and thus improving brain function.

Other Reasons for Dementia

- Alcoholism (Korsakoff's psychosis)
- Dementia from AIDS
- Lyme disease
- Parkinson's disease
- Huntington's disease

The problems associated with each of these dementias are similar to what has been discussed with Alzheimer's, only with a different cause. Here again we see that not everything that looks like Alzheimer's is truly Alzheimer's.

When thyroid hormone is given to a person who is low in it, any other illness that is causing troubling symptoms can sometimes be noticeably improved. It is not a lack of thyroid hormone that causes Parkinson's, Huntington's, Lyme disease, or AIDS. Instead, **the mental deficits from these conditions are worse if thyroid hormone is low**. Those symptoms can become greatly improved with normalization of the thyroid hormone levels.

A major psychiatric nursing textbook states: "An incorrect diagnosis for an elderly person experiencing dementia can lead to needless suffering, sometimes permanent impairment, or even death." (Frisch) Although dementia is generally considered an irreversible condition, it is our firm belief that *a great many elderly people are misdiagnosed*. What many of them have is *undiagnosed and untreated thyroid imbalance, causing an easily treatable dementia*.

> **A great many elderly people are misdiagnosed, especially when thyroid is the culprit.**

This condition can be remedied with very inexpensive, easily available, effective, and safe thyroid medicines. Treatment can reverse the condition partially or even completely.

Noreen Frisch, PhD, RN, and Lawrence Frisch, MD, write: "Severe memory deficits are not the result of normal aging. The first priority is to look for a simple, reversible cause." (Think thyroid.)

A major reason this problem is so frustrating is that *there can be thyroid hormone abnormalities in the brain that can escape detection* when measuring thyroid hormone levels in the bloodstream, our main method of diagnosis. (Joffe)

In some individuals, there is evidence that marginal hypothyroidism, if sustained for a long enough period, might produce irreversible cognitive dysfunction. (Haggerty) For this reason, it is crucial to test and treat early.

Autoimmune hypothyroidism frequently *coexists* with other auto-immune conditions. The newest research is showing that Alzheimer's may indeed be one of those autoimmune conditions.

> **Autoimmune thyroid imbalance might commonly coexist with many cases of true Alzheimer's.**

Recall that a coexistent thyroid problem makes any other illness worse.

This means it is even more imperative to give well-chosen Alzheimer's patients a chance for a trial of thyroid treatment, as long as such therapy can be safely and carefully monitored. Then, it may not matter so much whether thyroid imbalance or Alzheimer's is the true dementia diagnosis. Either way, there can be some thyroid improvement possible that would ordinarily have been missed.

More Fascinating Research on the Thyroid Brain

Before we had the ability to measure TSH directly, episodic slowing on EEGs was reported in subclinical hypothyroidism. (Fader) A significant percentage of the patients studied had definite cognitive decline. What could be the mechanism for some of these changes at the cellular level?

Dr. John Lowe has studied this relationship carefully. He suggests that inadequate thyroid hormone regulation of cell function is very likely to be associated with cognitive dysfunction through a variety of mechanisms.

Dr. Lowe feels that one of the important brain cell and blood vessel results of thyroid imbalance is increased density of alpha-adrenergic receptors and decreased density of beta-adrenergic receptors. The damage from these changes is subnormal brain cell metabolism, with reduced brain artery blood flow. (Lowe)

> **This is crucially important since the brain has a higher metabolic rate than other tissues.**

Hence, insufficient delivery of oxygen, glucose, and other metabolic substances in the brain is likely to result in a more severe dysfunction than it would in kidney or muscle. The dysfunction occurs because in the use of brain cells during thinking, metabolic rate is increased, as is the flow of blood through local vessels.

Inadequate thyroid hormone regulation impedes both of these physiological accompaniments of thinking. According to Dr. Lowe, cognitive dysfunctions mainly include deficits in memory and sustained concentration.

Another way of understanding this is:

> **The brain has a higher concentration of thyroid hormone receptors than most other tissues.**

When researchers measure the amount of messenger RNA in the various tissues, the brain has the highest concentration, especially in RNA that codes for thyroid receptors. (Oppenheimer)

Other researchers feel that hypothyroid people have impaired cognition related to a decrease in oxygen available for the brain's work. When a person is hypothyroid, the increased requirement of the brain cells for oxygen may not be met, contributing to the hypothyroid patient's cognitive impairment. (Schmidt)

This researcher feels that the gradations of hypothyroidism are mirrored in the gradations of impaired mental function. Research on the blood flow in hypothyroid patients showed that the cerebral blood flow was 38% below normal, while their oxygen consumption was reduced to 27% below normal.

Our Treatment Recommendations

The good news is that hypothyroid patients with impaired cognition can often return to normal with treatment of their hypothyroidism. This leads some researchers to believe that impaired cognition in hypothyroidism is the paradigm of physiological mental dysfunction. (Berne)

Over-the-Counter Remedies

The best natural remedy for people with cognitive and memory difficulties is the herbal remedy **guggulsterone**. This is a common treatment in the Ayurvedic pharmacopeia of medicines, less well known in the United States.

It has the beneficial effect of boosting thyroid function and responsiveness of the system to thyroid hormone. It is a component of many over-the-counter thyroid-boosting remedies sold at health food and vitamin stores. Lipotain, for instance, by Metagenics, has an excellent track record.

Treatment begins with **one tablet or capsule daily**. If after a week no improvement is noted, you can **increase to two daily**, both taken together in the morning. **Continue upward titration**. If, however, you have not had improvement and you are taking eight pills daily, this remedy is probably not for you.

Guggul, as it is sometimes called, works best in the presence of a strong antioxidant. The general antioxidant formulas sold at vitamin stores are often not effective enough for the kind of improvement needed by thyroid sufferers. We therefore recommend the nutraceutical versions, Oxygenics by Metagenics or Oraxinol by Xymogen. These are definitely more powerful and effective antioxidant formulas than are generally available over the counter.

When guggul and a good antioxidant are combined with the brain-boosting herbal medicine **gingko biloba**, or simply gingko, there are often additional benefits to health, including clear thinking and better memory.

Gingko is available by itself at many health food stores, but once again, a highly purified *standardized* version is available from the nutraceutical companies, combined with other helpful products. (GingkoRose and Ceralin by Metagenics are excellent. The Xymogen version, MemorAll, has been especially helpful to our patients.)

Prescription Treatment

In the absence of anxiety or adrenal mood disorders that sometimes accompany memory deficits, the cognitive treatment that has been most useful is **straight T3** thyroid hormone. This appears to be what is most lacking in brain dysfunction difficulties.

With either depression or especially anxiety, there is liable to be a strong *adrenal component*, usually an insufficiency of adrenal cortex hormone, such as cortisol. The use of a strong, quick-acting thyroid hormone, like T3, is less advisable in those easily worsened adrenal situations.

When dealing with memory loss or attention deficit, even with dementia, T3 would be the drug of choice (in the absence of cortisol limitations).

T3 can be administered as a prescription version, with the brand name **Cytomel**, or generic liothyronine. Good generic varieties are now available as well. Some people who need T3 do best with a timed-release product, available by prescription from a compounding pharmacy.

The initial starting dose should be small, on the order of 5 mcg per day or less. Keep this up for at least 2 weeks, before increasing to 10 mcg a day for the next 2 weeks. Thereafter, you can increase by an additional 5 mcg every 2 weeks, until a standard dose of 25 mcg is reached.

In the elderly population, these amounts should be scaled back a bit, with a close monitoring of the upward titration. Older people generally do better with less thyroid hormone than those who are younger.

Once particular dosage level is reached in terms of an initial response to therapy, or upon reaching the 25-mcg plateau, it would be best to let the patient stay with this dose for a period of 6 to 8 weeks, just to evaluate how much benefit is liable to accrue.

Resistance to Thyroid Hormone

Many people with cognitive difficulties have varying degrees of acquired resistance to thyroid hormone, even in standard doses. They *may need super physiologic doses* in order to get the same response as someone who does not have the same degree.

The issue of **resistance** to thyroid hormone is very much akin to the issue of insulin resistance. In these situations, **higher levels of the hormone are needed in order to have the same physiologic effect** as lower levels would have in most people.

If you do not receive the expected benefit from a standard dose of medicine, but do get benefit from a higher dose, resistance may be your situation. This can be tested by checking the level of Free T3 against Free T4.

If Free T4 is toward the higher end of the normal range, but Free T3 is toward the lower end, one may infer difficulty in converting T4 into T3 (active thyroid hormone).

This is simply one kind of resistance, but a very common one.

Testing Dilemmas

It is not always possible to use blood tests to initially diagnose or later monitor the therapy for a patient with resistance to thyroid hormone. Instead, what is needed is **a close monitoring of symptom reduction** and a keen observance to make sure there are no side effects to the therapy. This issue is of critical importance.

> **Far too often, the chance for effective thyroid treatment is missed because of *too rigid adherence* to supposedly accurate TSH blood tests.**

What we call "the tyranny of the test" forces people to fit within an artificial and often incorrect range of normal. In our view, **test results alone should *not* be used to make decisions about dosage adjustments**.

Our goal is to reach a beneficial effect. Peripheral blood values do not accurately assess whether the hormone therapy is beneficially affecting the central nervous system tissues. To do that, peripheral blood levels of T3 and T4 thyroid hormone (according to the standard tests) might have to be in the slightly high range.

If people have no physiological signs or symptoms of hyperthyroidism, and no hypermetabolism is noticed at all, then they are not likely to be truly hyperthyroid. This is especially true if they are finally—for the first time perhaps in years—becoming more normal in their cognitive function.

Although the above regimen described for you in this chapter has generally been the one we have found most effective, some Foggy types do better with other kinds of thyroid treatment. You may certainly want to try another thyroid treatment protocol if this chapter's recommendation is not as effective as you would like. You may consider trying treatments presented in Chapters 4, 5, 7, or 8. Keep trying until you feel your best!

Complementary Healing for Your Best Results

By Georjana Shames, LAc

You now have a sense of how the Chinese Medicine system of the Five Elements encompasses Fire, Earth, Metal, Water, and Wood—and that these Five Elements correspond within our new model of thyroid–mental health imbalances to Moody, Foggy, Needy, Sleepy, and Edgy. In this chapter, we delve into how the *Foggy* type of imbalance relates to the *Earth* element and *Spleen* Meridian.

The Spleen Meridian is responsible for transformation and transportation of nutrition within the body.

I like to describe its function as "extracting fuel from your food." When we are unable to properly extract fuel from the items we consume, that unused food becomes "Dampness," contributing to excess weight, tiredness, and the fuzzy thinking that leaves us confused.

In other words, someone who has poor digestion is fatigued (especially after eating) and hence plagued by attention deficit, confusion, or memory loss. These individuals definitely suffer from a deficiency of the Spleen Meridian.

The mental clarity aspect of the Spleen Meridian can be improved, however. In Chinese Medicine, any boost to the Spleen Meridian assists in quicker, more accurate mental functioning today, while also helping to ward off dementia later in life.

If you struggle with a Foggy mental state, becoming confused and forgetting names, dates, and tasks, it is easy to become discouraged. Fortunately, there are methods for restoring your mental clarity, including acupuncture, massaging specific points on yourself, and adding certain items to your diet to boost the Spleen Meridian and build the Blood.

CARING FOR YOURSELF

- Remember the tender area you found in Chapter 4, located near the ankle about 3 inches directly above the prominence of the medial malleolus? That point (**Spleen 6**) not only benefits the emotions but also assists with the Spleen Meridian's function of *transformation and transportation*. This makes it helpful for digestion, weight loss, and "foggy" thinking. **Note: Do not press this point if you are pregnant.**

- Another point to massage on yourself is located about 3 inches below the kneecap, 1 inch away from the shinbone on the lateral (outer) side. This is a very important point (**Stomach 36**) for strengthening the Spleen Meridian, resulting in *increased mental and physical stamina.*

RECIPES AND REMEDIES

Here is a delicious recipe for improving your mental clarity:

- In a medium saucepan, allow 3 cups of water to simmer before adding 2 small yams, thinly sliced, and a grated inch of fresh gingerroot.

- Cook for 10 minutes, then add 1 cup of goji berries (what we call *gou qi zi* in Chinese Medicine). Continue to simmer another 10 minutes.
- Goji berries resemble raisins but are a bright red color; they are sometimes referred to as "the Himalayan super-fruit" because of their high antioxidant content.
- This stir-fry (cooked in water, not oil, to avoid creating Dampness) makes two servings for a wonderful daily memory boost.
- **Avoid foods that make you feel more foggy and sluggish.** This could include dairy, fried foods, greasy foods, excess carbohydrates or sugars, or any food items that give you headaches or make you feel dazed and confused after eating. You can be allergy tested, something done at our medical clinic, so that you are more aware of which foods cause reactions that you seek to avoid.

STRATEGIES FOR MENTAL CLARITY

- **Moderate exercise** like speed walking, hiking, and gentle calisthenics, as well as getting fresh air and plenty of pure water each day, will improve your mental clarity. Naturally, this can be an excellent way for you to counter the effects of memory loss before they begin.
- A recent study found that **gentle exercise of 30 minutes' duration three times weekly** even improved the cognitive abilities of nursing home residents with dementia. (Stevens)
- You may also want to consider **increasing your memory-related tasks**, adding crossword puzzles, card games, Sudoku, and so forth.
- Help yourself out by **keeping important items** in the same place always. Your keys and cell phone, for instance, can be kept in the same pocket in your purse at all times, or perhaps have one bowl conveniently located by the front door of your house that holds your wallet, keys, cell phone, and grocery lists.

If you find yourself trying desperately to remember some critical piece of information, stop in your tracks and **take a minute to pause and breathe deeply**. This will help perfuse your brain with oxygen, keeping you calmer, so you can recall information without stress.

Good luck! Remember this is all part of the process of improving your mental clarity. It may not happen overnight, but certainly with the help of the suggestions from this book, you can feel more calm, cool, and collected, with clear thinking and a more robust memory.

THE BOTTOM LINE

There are many kinds of memory disorders, especially in the elderly. For a significant portion of them, **fixing an underlying thyroid problem can make a huge difference in how you feel and live your life**.

- ADD and ADHD can be relieved at times by adding thyroid hormone.
- Being foggy or weak-minded is *not* normal at any age.
- Thyroid treatment can help improve brain function in those with mild thyroid imbalances—and even in those with Alzheimer's.
- Normalizing thyroid hormone levels often helps brain function, because it normalizes blood pressure and lowers high cholesterol.
- The **brain has a higher metabolic rate** than other tissues. Thus, it is even more dependent on proper thyroid levels than other organs are.
- Difficulties in memory, focus, and concentration are often *symptoms of simple overactive or underactive thyroid*.
- Thyroid hormone resistance may require you to use slightly higher than "normal" medicine dosages to enable you to feel fully improved.
- A keen **awareness** of your own bodily responses is crucial to feeling your best.

RECOMMENDED ACTION PLAN

- For over-the-counter treatment of thyroid-related memory and focus issues, start first with **bioactive amounts of guggulsterone** (such as two daily Lipotain by Metagenics).
- Enhance the effectiveness of guggul's thyroid boosting with an extra-strong, well-tolerated **antioxidant** (such as one daily Oraxinol by Xymogen).
- If this is not fully helpful, add a trial of straight T3 prescription thyroid hormone (liothyronine). This can be brand name **Cytomel**, generic T3, or timed-release T3 from a compounding pharmacy.
- **Avoid foods that make you feel more foggy and sluggish.** This could include dairy, fried foods, greasy foods, excess carbohydrates or sugars, or any food items that give you headaches or make you feel dazed and confused after eating.

7

The SLEEPY Mind-Type

Relieve Insomnia, Narcolepsy, and Nonrefreshing Sleep

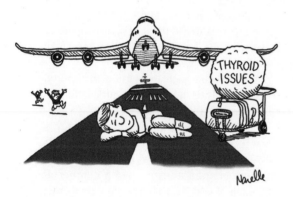

Andy's Story, Part 1

Andy Benson's successful life was falling apart. He was a tired 39-year-old neuroscientist, working at Duke Medical School. He consulted with us by phone after meeting us at a book-signing event we held at the Harvard Cooperative Bookstore, called the "Coop."

Andy complained of exhaustion, feeling awful and continually sleepy, wanting to be in bed all the time. He was tired and listless, which left him feeling totally unmotivated for anything in his life.

(continued)

Born in Omaha, he loved cold weather, feeling miserable when it was warm outside. He was always very bright, but by age 12 things became worse—plus, his grades suffered.

In high school he seemed to pull out of it and went on to college. There he did well academically, despite still feeling tired all the time. His medical checkups and psychological counseling sessions revealed no explanation for his ongoing fatigue. Special tests for chronic fatigue syndrome and Lyme disease were likewise normal.

He married a girl from college in his senior year, although he told us he always felt too flat to fall in love. After college he went to grad school in psychology and neuroscience, partly in search of an answer to his own health predicament.

He functioned well in his career, but still felt lousy. Always a night owl, he did not sleep well. The couple moved to Duke University, where they had a son and a daughter in short succession.

After a few more years, he was in the habit of returning home from work and falling onto the couch, barely able to arise. Mornings were even worse; he awakened feeling wiped out.

Andy responded to this fatigue with increasing irritability, especially in relating to his wife and kids. It became so difficult for her that she began threatening divorce.

Around the same time his wife was talking of divorce, his supervisors at work were threatening to let him go. Neither his doctors nor his experience as a neuroscientist was helpful in creating a solution for his exhaustion. He had already tried a number of different antidepressants, each of which had made him feel worse. All testing showed normal, leaving him feeling at his wit's end.

It turns out Andy is not alone.

What's at Stake?

Sleep disturbance or insomnia is the third most common patient complaint, ranking behind headaches and the common cold. Approximately 15% of the adult population in the United States has insomnia of significant enough severity to seek medical attention. More than 50% of elderly people have insomnia. (Kamel)

The consequences of untreated sleep problems may include significant emotional, behavioral, and cognitive dysfunction. (Nutter) Endocrine conditions affecting sleep are related to hyperthyroidism, menopause, the menstrual cycle, pregnancy, and hypogonadism in elderly men.

A number of medical conditions potentially can disturb sleep and need to be ruled out. These include chronic cardiac or lung disease, thyroid disease, gastroesophageal reflux, chronic pain, and other conditions. (Hertz)

According to the National Heart, Lung, and Blood Institute (NHLBI), a division of the National Institutes of Health in Bethesda, Maryland, the sleep problem is enormous. NHLBI estimated in 2007 that:

- 40 million Americans (1 in 6) have some degree of a sleep disorder.
- 30 million people (1 in 8) suffer from common insomnia.
- 18 million (1 in 15) are dealing with sleep apnea.
- Of that 18 million, 12 million have obstructive sleep apnea.
- 200,000 are believed to suffer from narcolepsy sleep disorder.
- Additionally, many thousands of others experience restless legs syndrome, severe jet lag, and circadian rhythm disorder.

There are many more statistics. What is important to understand is that with all these sleep-disordered people at work and in our environs, we are *all* more susceptible to accidents until we can ensure that more people are receiving the help they need. For many it can be as simple as balancing thyroid hormones.

Learning from Our Patients

Ever since we have been practicing in the thyroid arena, we have had patients tell us that their sleep was disturbed. Sometimes the sleep problem was the main reason for their coming to see us.

These were often people who knew they had a thyroid problem. They knew when it started. They received treatment for it, and most of their symptoms were resolved. But in some cases the sleep problem remained.

Others had come to our practice for a variety of other concerns, but invariably mentioned sleep disturbance as important. We found that sleep problems were a consistent abnormality in our thyroid patients.

It was striking how much improvement our sleep-disordered patients actually derived after receiving optimal thyroid care.

As many of their other symptoms were resolved, the sleep problem also began to improve. They initially spoke of a variety of nightly problems, including:

- Difficulty getting to sleep
- Frequent awakenings
- Waking at 3 a.m. and being unable to get back to sleep
- Waking unrefreshed, no matter how many hours they slept

The wide range of distress led us to believe that the *effect of thyroid imbalance on sleep patterns* was highly individualized.

It did not seem to matter whether the thyroid problem was high thyroid or low thyroid—both caused sleep disruption.

- The *high thyroid, or hyperthyroid, person* might be agitated and shaky during the day, a state (one could reason) that would be likely to interfere with the ability to fall asleep or to stay asleep at night.
- The *low thyroid, or hypothyroid, person*, on the other hand, talked often about being very tired, yet unable to fall asleep or stay asleep.

Since many glands work in tandem, a significant portion of our hypothyroid patients seemed to be producing *excess adrenaline* (made by the adrenal to compensate for low thyroid) in order to get through the day. As long as they were up and active, this excess adrenaline was barely noticeable.

When lying down to go to sleep, it was another story. With most muscle activity turned off, the patients now noticed the excess adrenaline in the form of continued thoughts, ruminations, planning, or worrying. At times they noticed it upon waking to adjust the covers or roll over. Then, the ruminations and anxiety would start, and they would not be able to get back to sleep.

In many patients with this particular profile, the relationship, life, or business events causing the worry did not change as treatment proceeded; only one thing changed.

What changed as they began taking thyroid hormone was their enhanced ability to get a good night's sleep.

Afterward, a large number of these patients were able to report that sleep was no longer a problem. The issue simply went away. They could go to sleep when they wanted. They slept well. They got up when they wanted, and felt refreshed.

This should have been the normal situation all along. For thyroid patients, however, a normal sleep pattern is often elusive. It generally returns when the thyroid imbalance is optimally corrected.

The picture was similar for people with hyperthyroidism. High thyroid patients also had sleep problems, which were directly related to their excessive thyroid levels. These, too, resolved well with good thyroid care. As hyperthyroid people, they of course needed to reduce their levels of the stimulating excessive thyroid hormone. When this was accomplished, they once again slept well.

Better than Prescription or Over-the-Counter Sleep Remedies

Who would have guessed that either hypothyroidism or hyperthyroidism was so involved with proper sleep? Sometimes a sleep problem is the only symptom of a thyroid imbalance. Treating it only as a sleep issue, without awareness of the underlying thyroid problem, can lead to only partial resolution.

A person may use a variety of natural remedies for better sleep, only to find them ineffective. Then they may switch to prescription remedies, only to find these to be partially effective and laden with side effects, including dependence and a 36% increased death risk. (Barclay)

The disrupted sleep may not sufficiently resolve until the underlying thyroid imbalance is fixed.

Many people were quite surprised to find out that their sleep issue was actually a thyroid issue. It so often occurred that we began to feel certain that thyroid problems and sleep problems were intertwined.

Cathryn's Story

Journalist and author Cathryn Jakobson Ramin, in her book *Carved in Sand*, describes the major change she experienced since coming to our clinic. In her words: "I just couldn't sleep, I couldn't sleep at all."

After a full evaluation with us, she was found to be low in thyroid hormone. We prescribed a small dose of the T3/T4 combo. Taking this personalized mix of thyroxines and thyronine each morning and night was quite successful for her over the long haul.

What she first noticed was that she really got her brain back, which is crucial for a writer. She joked that now, when she played "Race the Thesaurus," plugging a synonym of a word she was looking for into the search box, she could often produce the word even before the search engine found it. We considered this a positive step forward.

When she returned to our office after weeks of treatment, she informed us that she was sleeping a bit better. After a more lengthy involvement with hormone balancing, she now sleeps "fantastically," 7 hours a night, without waking up.

Thyroid and Sleep

Based on a wide variety of research projects exploring chemical mechanisms of sleep, here are some general conclusions from thyroid experts.

- Mary Shomon, amazingly dedicated patient advocate and prolific in all things thyroid, shared this: **"Problems with sleep are especially common in people with an overactive thyroid.** Symptoms can include difficulty falling asleep. Even after you do fall asleep, you may wake up frequently, and find it hard to get back to sleep. You may have insomnia and not be able to sleep at all. Because you are not reaching a deep sleep, you may wake up feeling tired and un-refreshed." (Shomon)

- Julia Ross, a dynamic and delightful colleague practicing near us, has this to say: **"You can't win any mood contests if you're losing sleep** on a regular basis. Sleep is a vital recharging process for both your mind and your body. . . . If you don't get enough sleep or don't sleep well, you'll suffer various physical consequences, but you'll also suffer emotionally." (Ross)

- In her book *The Mood Cure*, Ross suggests that the **three different kinds of thyroid malfunction (hypothyroidism, hyperthyroidism, and thyroiditis) could all affect sleep**. She also addresses sleep apnea, providing various nutritional remedies to help each kind of sleep disturbance, and others.

- According to Mark Starr, MD, thyroid clinician and author of *Hypothyroidism Type 2*, the idea of sleep being an issue for thyroid goes back as much as a hundred years ago. At that time, a famous endocrinologist, Dr. Hertoghe, the first of a long line of Hertoghe endocrinologists, suggested to advise medical students and fellow doctors: "When you encounter **significant ongoing somnolence or sleepiness, think of a possible deficiency of thyroid secretion.**"

- Dr. Starr further states, "The excitable effects of thyroid hormone in the synapses make it difficult for hyperthyroid patients to sleep, but **extreme sleepiness is the hallmark of hypothyroidism.**"

- According to endocrinologist and thyroid professor Ridha Arem, MD, "Abnormal sleep is in fact viewed as a major symptom of an abnormal thyroid." In his book *The Thyroid Solution*, Dr. Arem says, "**Patients can have brain hypothyroidism even though blood thyroid hormone levels are normal.**" (Arem)

- He writes, "Sleep disturbance will be part of a symptom profile that may lead physicians to think that there is a psychological illness present, such as depression, for instance, **when in actuality it is what most people would now call a physical illness, the actual lack of thyroid hormone from hypothyroidism.**"

- Glenn Rothfeld, MD, and Deborah Romaine published an intriguing book called *Thyroid Balance*, in which they state, "**The thyroid gland produces the hormones that regulate nearly every bodily function.**" Restorative sleep is one of those functions.

A Look at the Science

Scientists actually know that sleep is an altered state of consciousness that can be easily disrupted by an internal sensation or external stimulus. It is very different from simply turning off your laptop computer. When a computer is off, it is not functioning. The brain, however, our "bio-computer," works differently.

Actual sleep is a surprisingly active and dynamic state for humans as well as for other members of the animal kingdom. A great deal is happening whether people are dreaming and having a vivid nightmare or resting so peacefully that they will have no recollection of anything. Either way, the process is a complex, full, and very busy physiological state.

Extensive studies document that disruption of sleep adversely affects humans in a variety of ways. People need their sleep; when they don't get it, they start to behave poorly, feel poorly, and have undesirable health repercussions.

In fact, **ordinary unrelenting sleep deprivation has caused many people to go crazy.** In extraordinary circumstances it has been used as a method of torture. In addition, there is a syndrome called FFI (fatal familial insomnia), which causes the inability to enter deep sleep via destruction of cells in the relay center of the brain (thalamus). It is extremely hereditary, and those who suffer from it die from it.

Measuring Brain Activity

We now view sleep as a state of altered consciousness, rather than unconsciousness. Different levels of consciousness can be measured by simple electrical recordings made from the outer surface of the head.

Measuring electrical activity in the brain (nighttime EEG) reveals a standard pattern of complex and constantly flowing current waves all through the night. This is no simple "resting state." Something very important and intricate is taking place.

Just to give you a better idea of how delicate and fine-tuned this process actually is, we ask you to follow along on the journey through a typical night's sleep. As you do, just imagine how important it might be to have the right rate of thyroid metabolism in the brain.

- As you fall asleep, your brain waves slow down and become synchronized. You are entering Stage 1 of slow-wave sleep. As time passes, your brain waves become even slower and more synchronized.
- You then gradually go deeper into sleep, descending in order through Stages 2, 3, and 4. Stage 4 is known as *deep sleep.*
- At these deeper stages, muscle tone and muscle activities diminish, blood pressure decreases, and heart rate slows. You become more

difficult to arouse. This deep sleep is what younger people especially seem to need to feel restored. It is sorely missed when sleep
is insufficient.

- Oddly enough, the need for this kind of sleep, and the amount of
  time you will spend here, decreases as you get older. By age 60 not
  much time is spent in this stage at all.

- After roughly 70 to 80 minutes, you retrace your steps upward to
  lighter and lighter stages, and then proceed into rapid eye movement, or REM, sleep.

- This usually lasts for 20 minutes or so. The EEG brain waves
  become smaller and less synchronized, similar to the irregular and
  high-frequency beta waves of wakefulness. Your eyes are closed,
  but behind the lids they are moving around, as if watching things
  happen. You are now dreaming.

- Muscle tone at this point disappears, reflexes are inhibited, and
  brief contractions of the muscles can occur, but there is little organized movement of the body. This is thought to prevent us from
  physically acting out the movements being dreamed.

- During this time, the EEG shows a variety of wave patterns going
  from the visual cortex to the brain stem.

- After a varying period of REM sleep, the whole process just
  described is poised to repeat. This has been one sleep cycle.

- Descending once again deeper through the four stages, then
  going lighter, and then going into REM will constitute another
  sleep cycle.

- As the night progresses, you spend less time in deep sleep and more
  time in REM.

- Ideally you might have five cycles per night, and wake up delight-
  fully refreshed. If the alarm clock wakes you up during REM sleep,
  this is when dreams are often remembered.

Full health requires that this entire multistage process be completed,
with everything proceeding in proper order. Sleep is far more complex
than simply turning off an overheated motor to let it cool. Vital brain
activities are taking place that science is just beginning to understand.
One thing is clear: you definitely want to have a normal thyroid metabolic
drive for this important, intricate process.

The Thyroid Connection

Exactly how is the thyroid related to sleep? It is absolutely crucial and vitally important to have normal thyroid hormone balance to be able to sleep properly. Unbalanced thyroid regulation causes sleep disruption several different ways. Some of these mechanisms have been studied much more completely than others. Nevertheless, brief descriptions of a few examples will serve to illustrate the intimate relationship of thyroid hormone with the sleep cycle.

- Inadequate thyroid hormone can increase the density of alpha-adrenergic receptors, decreasing the density of beta-adrenergic receptors.

  — Increased alpha-receptor activity may induce a drowsy wakefulness and may inhibit the slow-wave non-REM sleep, or it may obstruct actual REM sleep at the time of dreaming.

  — Decreased beta-adrenergic activation may increase drowsy wakefulness and decrease REM sleep.

  — Either receptor change can explain hypothyroidism's association with a lack of sufficient Stage 4 sleep.

- Another mechanism is that the thyroid hormone inadequacy can result in uncomfortable **contraction of the muscles**. This may compress veins, decreasing the flow of metabolic waste products. These metabolic products may irritate the nerve endings. **This activation of nerves could result in uncomfortable signals to our central nervous system.**

- **Compression of the arteries** may reduce the supply of nutrients in the muscle cells, inducing mild deficiency contractures. The results may be the formation of uncomfortable **painful spots in the muscles**. This discomfort can enter the spinal cord and be transmitted to the brain, passing through the brain stem. While passing through the brain stem, these impulses of discomfort stimulate the **reticular activating system** of the brain stem, one place from which the initiation and continuation of sleep is thought to emanate.

Sleep Symptoms Can Be Either Cause or Effect

In this chapter we mainly discuss how altered hormone balance can interfere with normal sleep. The reverse, however, is also quite true. Disrupted sleep from some other cause, like the very common mechanical upper airway obstruction, can interfere with proper hormone balance.

Both *upper airway resistance syndrome* and *true sleep apnea* can alter your hormones. They can increase cortisol, lower leptin, raise hypocretin, and lower hypothalamus TRH, which lowers pituitary TSH, which lowers thyroid and interferes with the stomach's release of ghrelin, which helps control appetite.

> **Changes in any one of these can affect your glucose metabolism— and eventually your weight.**

Thus, some people may experience disturbed sleep as the *cause* of their thyroid problem. For that situation, we recommend reading the excellent book *Sleep, Interrupted* by Steven Park, MD, or visiting his website www.SleepInterrupted.com.

We have had good luck treating sleep issues that are the *result* of thyroid problems, but it can get complicated. Disturbed sleep from thyroid imbalance can easily result in its own set of nonthyroid symptoms, which can then merge with the original thyroid symptoms, often leading to a *confusing clinical picture that needs careful evaluation*.

> **Sleep disturbance from thyroid imbalance can complicate or worsen other signs and symptoms of high (or low) thyroid.**

With abnormal amounts of thyroid hormone, sleep disruption can occur and persist, despite otherwise optimal circumstances for sleep (such as familiar surroundings and your own comfortable bed). Moreover, it can often persist despite any number of sleep enhancers or medicines utilized as remedies.

Once again, we want to emphasize that either high or low thyroid can lead to deficiency of sleep, by stimulating the reticular activating system of the brain stem or by affecting ATP production.

As mentioned earlier, this sleep control area, when stimulated a certain way, will produce a greater alertness that can strongly interfere with sleep. This type of disturbance is more often seen in high thyroid.

Keep in mind that:

- *Mild hyper*thyroidism can cause people to **sleep lightly**.
- *Moderate hyper*thyroidism can cause **significant sleep disturbance**.
- *Severe hyper*thyroidism can cause **total lack of sleep and mania**.

Likewise, it may be interesting to note that:

- *Mild hypo*thyroidism can cause people **to sleep lightly**.
- *Moderate hypo*thyroidism can cause **significant sleep disturbance**.
- *Severe hypo*thyroidism can cause **continual sleep or coma**.

Changes in Serotonin

Another effect of hypothyroidism is alteration of serotonin excretion. As you may recall from Chapter 4, **serotonin** is a thyroid-dependent **brain transmitter chemical**, thought to be key in solving the riddle of depression. What does serotonin have to do with sleep? Plenty!

Our sleep mechanism—that elaborate, wonderful apparatus, so complex and so necessary for well-being—is maintained and controlled by a number of different hormones.

- The first arises starting in the afternoon, with gradually increasing levels of **melatonin**, reaching a peak around 10 p.m.
- Melatonin is produced in the pineal gland from serotonin. **Before you can have serotonin**, you must have **tryptophan**, a simple amino acid. Tryptophan becomes **serotonin**, then serotonin becomes **melatonin**.

As the brain perceives increasingly less daylight in the afternoons, there is an increased transformation of serotonin into melatonin. As this builds, it gradually induces you into the sleep cycle.

Having enough pineal gland melatonin is crucial. If you lack adequate serotonin, you may not be able to make enough melatonin.

Thyroid problems are known to affect these metabolic steps. In the broadest sense, not having enough thyroid hormone—as in low thyroid conditions—means the brain does not have enough T3 for proper production of serotonin.

- A number of studies suggest that a thyroid-inspired serotonin deficiency results in disturbed sleep. (Weinstock)
- It appears that serotonin deficiency can reduce slow-wave sleep as well as REM sleep. (Morgane)

One mechanism proposed to explain why certain **antidepressants** help people sleep when taken at night is that **they increase the concentration of key neurotransmitters in the central nervous system**. This nighttime antidepressant maneuver, so helpful in the general population, works less well in hypothyroid patients, unless they also take thyroid hormone.

It has thus been proposed that the underlying mechanism of the low serotonin level and sleep difficulty in hypothyroid patients is the **inadequate thyroid hormone regulation of the adrenergic genes, with an increase in alpha-adreno-receptors on the membranes of the serotonergic neurons**.

> **People with hypothyroid sleep disturbance really need an *increase in thyroid hormone*.**

In this light, taking a strong synthetic chemical sleeping pill for delicate thyroid hormone–related sleep problems can be akin to releasing a bull in a china shop. The sleeping pill maneuver temporarily helps, but for these patients, **thyroid is the real thing**.

Another interesting aspect of this biochemistry is that the very specific *thyroid-hormone-regulating enzyme*, called **5-prime-deiodinase**, is remarkably active in the pineal gland.

> **5-prime-deiodinase is the enzyme that converts transport thyroid hormone (T4) into active thyroid hormone (T3).**

Another compelling aspect of this thyroid-sleep connection is that **melatonin levels are found to correlate with a rise or fall in levels of TSH and T3**. (Soszynski) Many researchers are convinced of the thyroid's key role in the metabolism of melatonin. (Bals-Pratsch)

Special Sensitivities

Another underlying mechanism for how thyroid imbalance leads to sleep disturbance is in the area of **muscle weakness**. Weakness is an almost universal symptom of hypothyroidism. Weak muscles might affect oxygenation potential in various ways.

The slumped-over **posture** favored by many hypothyroid patients, which is due to weakness of spine muscles, might contribute to a less effective functioning of the diaphragm. The reduced effectiveness of the normal inspiration and expiration can easily result in suboptimal oxygenation of the blood, as well as sluggish digestion. (Schafer)

Another area of thyroid-related sleep disruption is reflected in **the ease of disturbance by external stimuli**. The senses and nerves of hypothyroid people are already irritated. They are more likely to be disturbed by external stimulation, such as extraneous noises in the home, than the average person is.

Normal people are able to deal with sounds, temperature changes, vibrations, or other kinds of stimuli, and bounce back from them to sleep. A **hypothyroid person is much more easily awakened** and will have more difficulty getting back to sleep. (Luden)

It should by now be abundantly clear that thyroid hormone is exquisitely involved in sleep. Sleep is actually a highly tuned, delicate combination of processes so complex and intricate that it requires all aspects of the system to be working properly. Any of this can easily be affected by something as profoundly disruptive as out-of-balance thyroid hormone, with accompanying changes in brain metabolic rate.

Andy's Story, Part 2

When we left Andy Benson, he was facing divorce and about to lose his job at Duke University. His constant "tiredness for no reason" was exacting an increasing toll on his life. No matter how much sleep he got, it was unrefreshing, leaving him increasingly less able to function well.

Medical workups and EEG sleep studies had revealed nothing, other than a vague decrease in Stage 4 sleep. A TSH test was "normal," so thyroid was not suspected. Unlike many sleep-deprived people, he did not have sleep apnea or upper airway resistance syndrome. No sleep supports or CPAP treatments had been of any benefit at all.

His medical doctors had suggested that with all tests and evaluations normal, it must be a psychological problem. Despite this recommendation, he had been totally unsuccessful with psychotherapy or antidepressants.

He tried using a variety of over-the-counter and prescription medications, with poor results. He tried different neurotransmitter boosters, as well as meditation, all to no avail. Some of these helped at the beginning, and then his reactions would worsen.

Eventually, he sought help from a well-known Harvard depression expert. This doctor did not want to treat him because he felt there must be some kind of hormonal issue complicating the case.

That was when Andy attended our *Thyroid Power* book signing, while visiting Boston. There, he acquired a new suspicion about the thyroid-sleep connection.

Andy first took the quick quiz on our website www.FeelingFFF.com and found symptom confirmation that he may indeed have a thyroid problem. He then called our office for a telephone coaching session. After evaluating his situation carefully, we recommended several additional thyroid tests.

One of these revealed the presence of thyroid antibodies. These had not been previously ordered because the TSH was so perfect. He now had a presumptive diagnosis of Hashimoto's autoimmune thyroiditis.

Based on this and our recommendations, he obtained from his doctor at Duke a prescription for the combination of both T3 and T4 thyroid hormone.

Here is the brief version of what happened: Andy was encouraged with some mild initial improvement. Eventually, his nighttime sleep started feeling much more restorative. His daytime activity became less lethargic. The grouchiness and irritability seemed to fade away. Everyone was pleased; both his marriage and his job were saved.

This story has a happy ending. Many others do not yet have such a favorable resolution. The rather common thyroid-sleep connection is all too often unsuspected. A higher index of suspicion for possible thyroid involvement would lead to better results.

An Even More Dramatic Sleep Problem

True *narcolepsy* is a rare disorder that causes **periods of extreme daytime sleepiness**, sometimes of sudden onset. It may be associated with muscle weakness as well. The most severe form involves people who can and do sometimes fall asleep in the middle of talking or eating. Most of the affected people report that they have trouble sleeping at night.

It is interesting to note that **narcolepsy may also cause cataplexy**, a sudden loss of muscle tone lasting a few seconds to a few minutes. Oddly, this is identical to what is seen when a normal person enters REM sleep.

Also associated with narcolepsy are super-**vivid dreams** when falling asleep or waking up that qualify as hallucinations. This may be caused by the rapid onset of REM sleep. A more severe aspect of this condition can be **sleep paralysis**, a situation that prevents a person from moving or speaking when either waking up or falling asleep.

This particular sleep difficulty is also intimately connected with thyroid imbalance. Like most thyroid issues, narcolepsy also seems to be autoimmune.

- In 2004, the British medical journal *Lancet* reported that Australian researchers had induced narcolepsy symptoms in animals by injecting them with antibodies from narcoleptic humans. This proved an immune connection.

- The autoimmune phenomenon is believed to be one reason for a lack of the chemical hypocretin. In the normal state this substance helps control levels of wakefulness. Narcoleptic individuals have low levels of hypocretin, as tested by measuring the fluid surrounding the spinal cord, obtained by spinal tap.

- It has been observed that low hypocretin narcoleptic men have altered settings of the pituitary-thyroid system, namely **abnormal TSH** levels. Scientists have confirmed that sleep onset can be correlated with changes in thyroid-stimulating hormone. (Kok)

We mention all this to demonstrate how thyroid issues can be involved with the severe disorders as well as the very mild ones.

Only some of the people with any kind of sleep condition have thyroid as a significant factor.

But, once you have determined that *your* sleep problem may be thyroid related, exactly what can you do about it?

Our Treatment Recommendations
Over-the-Counter Remedies

Our best recommendation for those having sleep difficulty due to thyroid issues is to **bring the system back into balance as gently as possible.**

- This may first involve use of gentle rebalancers, like **homeopathic remedies**. Keep in mind that homeopathic **remedies are not recommended for ongoing use.** Generally, you should stop taking them as soon as any improvement occurs. If you see no improvement after 2 weeks, stop anyway and move on to something else.
  - If the problem is **low thyroid**, then start with **Thyroidinum**, 6 or 12 potency (available through Boiron or Hyland's companies). If these products are not stocked by your local health food store, they should be able to order it for you. Dissolve *five pellets* under the tongue *three times daily for 2 weeks*, then stop.
  - For sleep disorders related to **high thyroid** levels, the **homeopathic** of choice is **Coffea Cruda**. Start with 6 or 12 potency. Take *five pellets* under the tongue *three times daily for 2 weeks* to assist sleep and to relieve agitation and sleep deprivation.

    Low-potency remedies like this are often available at health food stores or at homeopathic clinics. Stronger, higher-potency remedies are available from a homeopathic practitioner by consultation.
- If the above has not been helpful, the next thing to try is a specific actual **thyroid function booster**. Some combination thyroid remedies are particularly effective. We recommend two tablets each morning of **Thyrosol** by Metagenics, or four capsules each morning of **MedCaps T3** by Xymogen.
- **General herbal sleep medicines** can be exceptionally helpful for slumber difficulties due to thyroid imbalance. **Valerian root, passionflower, hops, lady's slipper**, and **orange peel** work well,

providing beneficial support to both the thyroid and the sleep system. Individually or as a combination, try two to four 00-size capsules at bedtime.

- **Skullcap** herb provides slower onset and lasts longer than the herbs listed above. It can strengthen your sleep regimen for a longer night's rest. Use the same dose and number as the herbs above.

- Metagenics also has a product called **MyoCalm P.M.**, which helps with muscle aches and pains, using calcium and magnesium, combined with passionflower, valerian, hops, and lemon balm as an effective herbal combo. Take three to four tablets at bedtime.

- An alternative to these is the Xymogen formula **Sedalin**, which combines two extraordinarily useful herbs, magnolia and ziziphus, for help in achieving a more normal sleep cycle.

- People who have had thyroid-related sleep difficulties are encouraged to not only try herbal sleep aids and thyroid hormone enhancers but also take the **amino acid L-tryptophan**. This is a serotonin precursor (available from practitioners) to help induce nighttime sleep more easily.

- More readily available to larger numbers of people is the tryptophan precursor called 5-hydroxytryptophan, or **5-HTP**, which can be purchased at most health food and vitamin stores. One or two 100-mg capsules taken at bedtime increases tryptophan levels, which then increases serotonin levels, helping you to fall asleep comfortably and to stay asleep longer.

    It is to be noted that 5-HTP is not an herbal remedy, though often mixed with herbs to good advantage. This is an amino acid, a precursor to serotonin. Extra 5-HTP at night has been a time-honored maneuver to lull the mental apparatus into a more comfortable sleep. It also helps people to sleep longer at a time. Many people in our practice are having positive results using it an hour before bedtime. It is highly recommended *not* to take 5-HTP while using SSRI antidepressants.

- **Somnolin** (by Metagenics) is a combination of vitamin B_6, folate, B_{12}, 5-HTP, and another calming amino acid, theanine. This multi-pronged approach is a stronger aid to sleep.

- Another nonherbal approach to better sleep is **melatonin** itself. If you have thyroid-related melatonin deficiency, 1 to 2 mg of this substance at bedtime is quite useful and surprisingly effective. As you age, natural levels of melatonin are often too low for supporting a quick onset and long duration of comfortable sleep. If you are in this category, melatonin at bedtime can be extremely helpful.

Keep in mind that *more than 1 mg* at night regularly can be associated with headache and depression as **side effects**. Be wary of melatonin products available at 5 mg or higher. In our view, this is excessive for regular intervention in an ongoing sleep problem.

Prescription Medicine

Because our delicately balanced and crucially important sleep mechanism is so finely tuned, it is often helped by carefully combining T3 and T4 hormones. T3 alone could be too stimulating; T4 alone could be less effective.

An *individualized* combination of T3 and T4 has been found to be most effective for sleep.

The best way to do personalized combination therapy is with *two bottles*, each with a different kind of thyroid hormone medicine:

- One with standard off-the-shelf **T3** tablets (brand Cytomel or generic liothyronine)
- The other with standard off-the-shelf **T4** tablets (brand Synthroid or generic levothyroxine)

The reason it might be best *not to have a fixed combination* of T3 and T4 all in one pill is that some people seem to need more of one kind of thyroid and less of the other. In those cases, it can be quite useful to adjust each of the two types of hormone individually.

Our Office Protocol

- We start with levothyroxine (T4), usually at 25 mcg per day in the morning.
- After 2 weeks we continue the above, now adding one-half of a 5-mcg tablet of T3 each day, also in the morning.
- Then we follow the patient's progress to see if this combination improves sleep over the next couple of weeks.

- If the patient feels too stimulated during the day and has more difficulty falling asleep, then we reduce the amount of T3.
- If the patient is actually getting some benefit in sleep but is feeling sluggish during the day, we increase the amount of T3.
- The T4 can later be increased from 25 to 50 mcg per day, if and when initial progress starts to recede. T3 can be increased from one-half pill to one or eventually two pills daily, if needed. We then advise staying at these doses for a couple of months before reevaluating.
- This amount of T3 and T4 generally yields a very good response.
- Again, the **titration is made based on the patient's symptoms**, while we also monitor from various blood tests drawn at intervals.

Many patients whose main difficulty is thyroid-disturbed sleep seem to feel best at a TSH level around 1.0, at which they derive adequate hormone support without being overstimulated.

It should also be noted that **bringing the T3 and T4 levels into mid-normal range is just the beginning**. The kind of permanent improvement we are seeking generally continues to build over the course of months, once the proper amount of thyroid medicine has been achieved. During this buildup phase, it is typically advisable to continue any previously prescribed drugs for sleep.

Later, **many of our patients find they can wean off other sleep medicines after optimal thyroid balance has been restored**. Most of them are quite pleased to be free of the high cost and uncomfortable side effects of Ambien, Sonata, or Lunesta. They now can hardly believe what extreme measures were required previously just to get a normal night's sleep. After caring for the thyroid, many aspects of their lives change for the better.

The bottom line . . .

Are we saying that everyone with any sleep problem should consider taking prescription thyroid hormone? The answer is *no*, of course not.

- If you experience *persistent problems with sleep*, have your **thyroid status evaluated carefully**.
- If your *thyroid tests show abnormality*, you deserve **treatment**.

- If, instead, your tests are normal, but you have compelling symptoms, related illness, family history, or physical signs of thyroid imbalance, you may still deserve thyroid treatment.
- In this case, however, it is called a "trial."

A practitioner-monitored trial of thyroid medicine in standard doses is quite **safe**. If you notice no improvement after a month on prescription medicine, then simply stop the trial. No big deal.

On the other hand, **if definite improvement is noted, then you have a life-changing diagnosis**. Thyroid medicine will not help any condition except a thyroid imbalance. If you are significantly improved, keep taking the medicine. Doing so is no longer a trial, but now is appropriate treatment for a newly diagnosed condition—thyroid imbalance.

Finally, we once again recommend that if the above treatment maneuvers are not helpful, please consider utilizing a different protocol, as presented in Chapter 4, 5, 6, or 8.

Although the T3/T4 combo regimen described in this chapter has been generally effective for thyroid-related sleep problems, some people do better with a different regimen. There are many kinds of prescription thyroid treatments.

If our initial recommendations in this chapter are not as effective as you would like, you are encouraged to try another good regimen. Whichever approach you choose, be sure to include some of the suggestions below.

Complementary Healing for Your Best Results

By Georjana Shames, LAc

In my model of the Five Elements of Traditional Chinese Medicine, the Sleepy type of suspected thyroid imbalance would correspond to the **Kidney Meridian**. In Chinese Medicine, the Kidney Meridian is considered the *root of the body's energy.*

You can imagine that a person who constantly feels fatigued, becomes tired after little exertion, awakens in the morning not refreshed after a night of poor sleep, and wants to nap often, suffers from Kidney Meridian deficiency.

The Kidney Meridian actually has two pertinent aspects, both of which relate to the Sleepy type of person.

- The Kidney Yang aspect can be thought of as the fuel for the body, like gasoline fueling a car's engine.
- The Kidney Yin aspect can be thought of as a relaxant for the body, like coolant for the car's engine.

Remember that your car runs successfully only with adequate supply of both gasoline and coolant. If fuel is in short supply, the car will sputter to a halt. If there is too little coolant, the car will still run but may begin to overheat, allowing vital components to burn out.

Sometimes a person is running low on one or the other. For many patients there is a **deficiency of both the Yin and the Yang**. This means they feel exhausted during the day, but cannot get good sleep at night.

It can be a vicious cycle: insomnia from Yin deficiency depletes the Yang energy, and deficient Yang energy triggers an attempt to compensate by burning through the Yin energy. Any Kidney imbalance affects not only the **physical stamina but also the mental state**, as evidenced by the quote "Harmony between the Kidneys and Heart is one of the prerequisites for a peaceful spirit." (Deadman)

Fortunately, there are methods of nourishing the Yin and strengthening the Yang of the Kidney Meridian. Acupressure points, dietetic suggestions, exercises, and a sustainable lifestyle are all part of restoring health to the depleted Kidney Meridian.

CARING FOR YOURSELF

- Locate the tender area on the inner ankle midway between the prominent bone of the medial malleolus and the Achilles tendon, which runs down the back of the ankle. This spot (called Kidney 3) is the source point of energy for the Kidney Meridian and is an excellent one to massage on yourself whenever you are feeling fatigued.
- Now locate the spot in the middle of the sole of the foot, between the second and third metatarsal bones, about one-third the distance from the base of the second toe to the heel. This area can be most easily found with the foot flexed, which reveals a depression in the bottom of

the sole. This point (called Kidney 1) calms the spirit and descends the Yang energy, so it is ideal to massage just before bedtime.

• If you tend toward insomnia, massage this point on first one foot then the other, for a total of 2 minutes each foot. Some people find that a little oil for the soles of the feet, such as soothing lavender-scented massage oil, is a beneficial addition to this before-bed routine.

RECIPES AND REMEDIES
A recipe containing foods and herbs to strengthen the Kidney Meridian for energy during the day and improved sleep at night would be hearty and very nourishing.

• Start by making a beef soup, simmering a large pot half full of water and placing in it 4 servings of beef chunks and the actual bovine bones to simmer for $\frac{1}{2}$ hour to infuse marrow into the soup stock.

• Remove the bones. Add 1 yam thinly sliced, 4 chopped carrots, and 2 inches of grated gingerroot. Allow this to cook another 10 minutes, adding salt to taste. Salt can be beneficial to the Kidney Meridian, as long as high blood pressure is not an issue for you.

• Serve the soup hot with a sprinkling of black sesame seeds.

EXCELLENT EXERCISE
Many different types of exercise benefit the Kidney Meridian, as long as you remember not to overexert yourself. Exercise builds energy, but you must start with a little energy first to actually reap the benefits of exercise. Otherwise you run the risk of exhausting yourself.

Begin with gentle stretching or a slow type of martial art like tai chi, and work up to more aerobic activities, as you are able. Videos on the gentle practices of qigong might well benefit you, as this form of exercise is designed to help nourish the energy within the various meridians.

Later, consider moderate or even vigorous bicycling, swimming, or jogging, but not to excess.

Remember to rest the body and the mind; more regular sleep and stamina will follow.

Finding the balance of a sustainable lifestyle is paramount for the Kidney Meridian, and it is an individual pursuit. You and only you can truly cultivate that for yourself.

It can be helpful to have affirmations to serve as reminders for that effort, something along the lines of *"All things in moderation"* or *"Balance is the key to my health."*

THE BOTTOM LINE

- Around 15% of the US population has insomnia, 50% of the elderly.
- Forty million Americans (1 in 6) have some type of sleep disorder.
- Our sleep-disordered patients derive great benefit from better thyroid care.
- The wide range of effects of *low or high thyroid* on sleep patterns is very personal and highly individualized.
- Most patients felt significant relief using just thyroid hormone.
- Inadequate thyroid hormone increases the density of alpha-adrenergic receptors, decreasing beta-adrenergic receptors.
- Thyroid hormone imbalance can result in uncomfortable contraction of the muscles, impacting nearby nerves and sending stimulation to the upper brain stem's sleep center, called the reticular activating system.
- Compression of the arteries may reduce the supply of nutrients in the muscle cells, inducing mild deficiency contractures, with the formation of uncomfortable painful spots in muscles.
- Upper airway resistance syndrome and true sleep apnea can alter your hormones as well as your sleep.
- Sleep disturbance from thyroid imbalance can complicate or worsen other signs and symptoms of high or low thyroid.
- A number of studies suggest that a thyroid-inspired serotonin deficiency results in disturbed sleep.
- Melatonin levels correlate with rise or fall in TSH and T3 levels.
- Many **sleep-testing abnormalities** can be symptomatic of underlying thyroid imbalance.
- Any **Kidney Meridian imbalance** affects not only physical stamina but also mental state.
- Remember to **rest** body and mind; more regular sleep and stamina will follow.
- **Balance** is a key to health.

RECOMMENDED ACTION PLAN

For over-the-counter treatment of thyroid-related sleep problems:

- If the problem is **low thyroid**, start with the homeopathic remedy **Thyroidinum**, 6 or 12 C or X potency, available at health stores. Take *five pellets* under the tongue *daily for a week or two*, then stop.

- **For high thyroid** levels, the homeopathic of choice is **Coffea Cruda**. Start with 6 or 12 potency. Take *five pellets* under the tongue *three times daily.*

- If the homeopathic remedies are not successful, you can then progress to a **thyroid function booster**, if needed. These include Thyrosol or MedCaps T3.

- **Herbal sleep products** known to help include valerian root, passionflower, hops, lady's slipper, and orange peel. Add skullcap for longer sleep.

- **MyoCalm P.M.** helps with muscle aches and pains at night.

- **Sedalin** combines two extraordinarily useful herbs, magnolia and ziziphus, for help in achieving a more normal sleep cycle.

- The **amino acid** L-tryptophan is a serotonin precursor (available from practitioners) to help induce nighttime sleep.

- More easily available and extremely helpful is the tryptophan precursor called **5-hydroxytryptophan (5-HTP)**.

- Somnolin is a combination of vitamin B_6, folate, B_{12}, 5-HTP, and another calming amino acid, **theanine**.

- If you have thyroid-related melatonin deficiency, 1 or 2 mg of **melatonin** at bedtime is quite useful for sleep.

  Then, if needed:

- Add a trial of **prescription T3/T4** combo from a qualified practitioner.

- T3 alone could be too stimulating; T4 alone could be less effective. In our office, an **individualized combination of T3 and T4** has been found to be the most effective for sleep.

- This is best accomplished with *2 separate bottles* of medicine: one of T4 (levothyroxine), the other of T3 (liothyronine).

8

The NEEDY Mind-Type

Recover from Eating Disorders, Substance Abuse, and Addiction

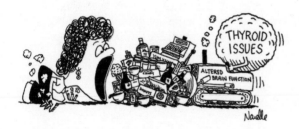

Maria's Story, Part 1

Maria was despondent. Her dream of becoming the first in her family to graduate college was rapidly unraveling. For months, she had secretly been starving herself, trying to look like her high school friends.

Maria, however, came from a family of larger women, several of whom had thyroid problems. Her anorexia was now at the stage where her electrolytes were severely off balance, causing nausea, dizziness, headaches, inability to sleep, fainting spells, shakiness, depression, and generalized weakness. She just felt awful and could not even function.

Months of starvation and throwing up had left her teeth

(continued)

damaged and her esophagus irritated. In fact, her entire digestive system was off-kilter. She became depressed, irritable, anxious, and fearful—doubting whether she could actually pull off this dream that had motivated her for so long.

With several college interviews looming, Maria realized she had to do something to get herself back in balance. Her desire to be thinner had become a serious barrier, threatening to stand between her and her goals of entry into college and eventual acceptance into law school.

She did not want to let her father down. He had always wanted one of his children to be a college graduate. He had brought the family into the United States 10 years before from the Mexican state of Michoacán.

For several generations in Mexico, their family had owned a little store outside a small town. Now, living in a big city had forced them to change many of their cultural ways.

Maria was a victim of cultural forces as well as physiological ones. The women in her family grew plump not just because of their rich diet but also because of a genetic tendency toward autoimmune thyroid problems.

No one in her family had ever been treated for this condition, even though it had been passed down for generations. No one, as far as Maria knew, had attempted to handle this bodily dilemma with starving or purging.

This new method was typically American, something she learned from her classmates in high school. For Maria, it started as a novelty; before long it became a coping mechanism. Soon it progressed into a compulsion and then an addiction.

Maria felt convinced that her starvation and bulimia were a necessity for her to get through her life. Without this behavior, she experienced extreme tension and preoccupation with maintaining her body image.

The throwing up not only kept her weight in check, but also seemed to relieve her anxiety. This ritual continued in secret, hidden from everyone, including her friends and family. Now she was headed for a crash.

What's at Stake?

Maria's *bulimia* is one type of eating disorder. Over 5 million Americans, mostly young women, have some form of this general malady. On US college campuses, especially in sororities, it is alarmingly prevalent. But just to be clear, it is definitely a worldwide problem.

This is just one part of the much larger worldwide problem known as addiction. Drug abuse and other addictive behaviors are a major burden to society. Estimates of the total annual costs of substance abuse in the United States—including health- and crime-related costs as well as losses in productivity—exceed $500 billion annually. (NIH)

Staggering as these numbers are, however, they do not fully describe the breadth of deleterious public health—and safety—implications, which include family disintegration, loss of employment, failure in school, and domestic violence, child abuse, and other crimes.

Eating disorders are particularly severe illnesses. Education and productivity are often cut short. Jobs and relationships are ruined. Disability and death are more commonly seen with these conditions than with many other diseases. Treatment, often involving hospitalization, is difficult and lengthy. Relapses are frequent, with eventual recovery rates disappointing. People who live but do not fully recover have a terrible life.

Worst of all for the treating practitioner, eating disorders represent a type of illness whose cause is largely unknown. The most that doctors can tell you is that these conditions share certain risk factors and personality traits:

- Abnormal onset of menstruation
- Low self-esteem and strong need for acceptance
- Home environment or career that emphasizes thinness
- Strict parenting with strong emphasis on physical attractiveness
- Peer group focus on and teasing about weight and dieting

Two Main Types of Eating Disorders

Bulimia nervosa consists of binge eating followed by compensatory efforts to minimize weight gain. The person who suffers this condition is characterized by a sense of dreadful loss of control during episodes, with concomitant remorse and low self-esteem. (Frisch)

THERE ARE TWO TYPES OF BULIMIA:

1. Purging type—regularly engages in self-induced vomiting or misuse of laxatives.

2.   Nonpurging type—tries to compensate for excessive food intake with excessive exercise or outright fasting from time to time.

Anorexia nervosa is characterized by a refusal to maintain a minimally normal body weight, along with an intense fear of gaining weight.

THERE ARE TWO TYPES OF ANOREXIA:

1.   Restricting type—weight loss usually accomplished by calorie restrictions, at times restricting all intake, often restricting all dietary fat.
2.   Purging type—excessive use of laxatives and diuretics. This condition is frequently characterized by a major effort on the part of patients to frustrate practitioner efforts to help them.

It is not enough to define and categorize these conditions. It would be better to be able to treat them effectively—and even better still to prevent them altogether. Learning a bit more about them might help.

Our Clinical Experiences

Some eating disorder risk factors seem similar to those of thyroid.

- They are both illnesses somehow related to the onset of puberty.
- They both run in families.
- They are both much more common in females.
- They both have strong psychological connections.

Could thyroid possibly be involved in eating disorders?

That question began to surface for us when our clinic signed on as medical backup to Recovery Systems of Mill Valley, a California eating disorder facility where the psychotherapist Julia Ross utilizes not only psychotherapy but also nutritional balancing of brain chemistry.

Her approach involves treating the blood sugar and neurotransmitter imbalances that contribute to anxiety and emotional eating. Sensible food intake, treatment of yeast overgrowth, boosting of fatty acid levels, and restoration of amino acid reserve are some of the components of this program. The goal is to evaluate and improve any aspects of metabolism that could contribute to food or substance addiction.

When Dr. Rich Shames started seeing the Recovery Systems clients, he was struck by how frequently women with an eating disorder had a family history of thyroid problems. Sometimes the patients themselves had been diagnosed with a thyroid problem in the past, often being told it had resolved and no longer needed treatment.

Previous to that time, his regular general practice would have a thyroid case only occasionally. But now, in Julia Ross's recovery population, thyroid problems were the norm. What was the connection?

We knew as clinicians that the body's *physical* functions depend upon a delicate balance of a great many specific chemicals, especially the powerful hormones. *Mental* function had more recently been shown to be the same. But what could be the actual involvement of thyroid hormone dysfunction in eating disorders?

It certainly seemed possible that severe dieting, as many of these women had done, may have triggered a mechanism that could have affected the thyroid. That was an interesting theory, but the medical history belied it. Most often the thyroid problems came long before the eating disorder.

In her book *The Diet Cure,* Julia Ross writes: "I've never met people who try harder at anything than the people that come to my clinic for help with eating issues. Over the years I've seen some of them immediately lose plenty of weight by following my diet and nutritional program. But—a great many others either lost weight very slowly, or not at all. They were frustrated to be eating and exercising so well, with little or no weight loss. Possibly their thyroid was part of the problem." (Ross)

Ross had by then claimed a 20-year history with this particular type of client. She has seen large numbers of people who keep their calories to a minimum, who exercise vigorously on a daily basis, and yet cannot seem to lose any weight at all. The doctors tell them that they are not trying hard enough. Yet these people chronically undereat and overexercise, since normal diets and sensible workouts cause them continued weight gain.

The research shows that fully half of people entering weight-loss programs do not overeat. Even good programs are often unsuccessful for certain people, until previously undiagnosed thyroid problems are treated.

The dropout rate for eating disorder programs without rigorous thyroid intervention can be more than 85%, as people often feel awful when detoxifying with sluggish eliminatory function. People are also terribly discouraged, and demoralized, due in part to the depression effect from apparently sluggish metabolism.

For many of these people, the thyroid is the culprit. Identifying and correcting low-functioning thyroid can make all the difference.

Endocrinology professor Ridha Arem, MD, says in his popular book *The Thyroid Solution* that underactive thyroid often exerts its influence through what is medically referred to as "atypical depression." (Arem)

Atypical depression is a form of chronic depression, commonly experienced by people with underactive thyroid. This patient can be occasionally cheered, but the improvement is short lived. She soon slips back into a depressive state, within hours or days afterward.

Symptoms may be mild or severe, but a big part of this particular profile is its relationship to sluggish metabolism. This is thought to be due to the underlying physical problem of having a low thyroid condition. In other words, according to Dr. Arem, **thyroid plays a major role in regulating overall eating behavior**. This was also our conclusion from Richard's monitoring of Julia Ross's recovery patients.

As medical backup to the Recovery Systems clinic, we also discovered that a great many other addictive behaviors and substance abuse issues seemed to be thyroid related.

In these people, the attempted correction of their problem could hardly begin to take place, and certainly could not improve, until the underlying thyroid problem was resolved. Often this required the addition of an appropriate amount and kind of thyroid medicine.

A Look at the Science

It has been known for well over 30 years that **an excess or deficiency of thyroid hormone alters** levels of endorphin, adrenaline, GABA, and serotonin. These **chemicals help control eating** behavior. (Gambert)

Furthermore, the thyroid hormone has a direct effect on the appetite centers of the brain. An **excess of thyroid hormone in the brain** could cause the person **to eat more often** and to select carbohydrates rather than other types of food. (Donhoffer)

Even a mild low thyroid condition, called low-grade hypo-thyroidism, can be a significant factor in weight problems. In 2009, an important research study showed that **very mild hypothyroidism**, even with officially "normal" blood ranges, **is highly associated with obesity.**

It should also be noted that if *excess* thyroid hormone has disturbed the appetite center, the **disturbance might persist** even long after the thyroid function has been corrected. Once someone previously hyperthyroid is treated, there can be residual effects while returning to a normal state, including increased appetite and increased caloric intake.

Endorphin, noradrenaline, leptin, and serotonin are all **biochemicals** that are **heavily impacted by thyroid hormone levels.** They all play a key role in eating behavior and eating disorders. According to Mark Hyman, MD, people treated for thyroid imbalance with standard blood testing showing normal levels can still suffer from severe symptoms in this area and may benefit greatly from further thyroid treatment.

Dr. Hyman also suggests that many patients hope that the answer to their weight challenge is slow metabolism. While not true for all, it can be true—according to Dr. Hyman—in one in five women. These are women who definitely should be checked for hypothyroidism. Not doing so more often is a failure of modern medical practice.

Doctors need to check more often, and patients need to help by being aware of this thyroid possibility in themselves.

Screaming to Be Understood

Another wonderful resource for women and girls facing these challenges is the well-researched book by Elizabeth Lee Vliet, MD, *Screaming to Be Heard: Hormonal Connections Women Suspect and Doctors Ignore.* While she realizes she is preaching to the choir in writing to women about their hormonal connections, her work is about hormonal effects on the brain and body systems, and how these interact with metabolic and nervous systems.

Dr. Vliet suggests that if you wish to get tested for thyroid, all too often with women, the clinical problems of weight and eating disorders may be present, but thyroid testing is normal. "Keep persisting," she says.

> **Thyroid antibody testing may be the solution to proving this often overlooked and under-considered connection to weight and eating disorders.**

With elevated antibodies having helped to make a diagnosis, prescription thyroid medicine can be amazingly helpful. She provides the example of a woman who had increased cravings and marked loss of energy for years. No amount of exercise would help.

Dr. Vliet then tested her thyroid antibodies and found "striking" abnormality on one of the patient's antibody tests, showing 1,660 (normal range 0 to 35). Even though she had normal blood results for TSH, her antibodies revealed the problem.

The doctor felt that the thyroglobulin antibody was acting as some sort of binding site blocking agent, preventing the thyroid from working properly, leaving the patient in a very unpleasant clinical condition. With the addition of thyroid hormone to overpower the abnormality, the patient later told the doctor she was finally back to her old self.

Dr. Vliet discusses how very important it is for readers to pay attention to what are clearly brain function changes. She provides the example of a person who for 30 years was doing fine, then began to have a strange relationship with food. She felt that the patient might possibly be experiencing a brain alteration, because "the brain is exquisitely dependent upon normal balance for optimal function . . ."

She furthermore explains how a great many international studies of brain function have recently shown that *changes in neurotransmitters, especially serotonin,* are an underlying *cause of eating disorders* in so many women.

This crucial connection shows up in her patient questionnaires, where she now asks, "Has your body and scalp hair become thin and fine, or are you losing a lot of hair?" What could this possibly have to do with eating disorders? A lot! This symptom is a key telltale sign of hidden thyroid imbalance.

In the decade following Dr. Vliet's book publication, the researchers were able to confirm with greater certainty a number of major assertions she was proposing. The work underpinning this field is related to brain metabolism.

Metabolism is the sum of all chemical reactions that occur inside the cells of that particular organ. Biochemically, this is a carefully regulated system of pathways, each contributing to activities that every tissue must carry out.

Considering eating disorders or other addictions, brain function is one of many systems (physical and mental) potentially directly regulated by the chemical process inside the cells known as metabolism. A major determiner as to whether or not the brain's metabolism functions properly is *thyroid hormone*.

Beyond Eating Disorders

It should now be apparent that correctly treating a thyroid gland that has previously been either deficient or excessive can make all the difference between normal eating behavior and exaggerated cravings or compulsions.

Eating disorders are only **one kind of craving** related to thyroid imbalance. There are a number of others:

- **Substance addictions**—caffeine, alcohol, tobacco, or sugar
- Abuse of prescribed medications, such as for pain
- Addiction to narcotic or hallucinogenic substances (street drugs)

All these and more can be significantly impacted by the balance or imbalance of thyroid.

To Feel Normal

There appear to be some people with sluggish metabolisms who have a defective ability to stimulate their own brain pleasure centers with ordinary activities of life.

As a result of this deficiency, **they require the more intense stimulation of substances or drugs.** This is another example of how altered thyroid brain function and addictive behavior may be linked.

Julia Ross discusses how people can enter the addictive zone. A great many of her addicted clients tell her that they didn't use these drugs in order to get high; they "just wanted to feel normal." They were uncomfortable enough to self-medicate in desperate efforts to feel like other people seemed to feel.

She had first thought that many of these addicts came from stressful childhoods that may have depleted their brain chemicals. She recalls being shocked reading studies showing that children of nonalcoholic biological parents who were adopted into alcoholic families did not tend to become alcoholic themselves. Children born to alcoholic biological parents adopted by nonalcoholic parents often became addicted.

The drive to addiction seems clearly related to inherited brain chemistry, quite possibly via the thyroid connection.

One more thought on genetic predisposition: a study in the year 2000 reported that *twins* had a tendency to share occurrence of certain eating disorders, such as anorexia, bulimia, or obesity. Evidence suggests there is an association between the genetic factors responsible for proper brain metabolism and susceptibility to eating disorders.

If genetic factors are involved, here is something to consider:

Thyroid is one of the most inherited of all illnesses.

One might safely suppose that relatives of people with thyroid disorders might show a genetic predisposition to having this condition. They deserve to be checked fully and to have this condition treated in order to bring their metabolic rates into normal range. (Ilias)

The Need to "Fix" a Sluggish Brain

In her book *The Mood Cure,* Ross says: "**The need for stimulants often signals a thyroid problem.** Stimulant drugs or uppers can do some of the things that thyroid is supposed to do. It speeds up metabolism in the body and the brain." **When we are low thyroid or underthrottled, we crave energy.**

People who need metabolic slowing down often gravitate to downers. One of the primary reasons some people may get addicted to alcohol is that their blood sugar tends to drop too low too often, a side effect of thyroid-related alcohol metabolism. Alcohol frequently makes these individuals so hypoglycemic that they *need* another drink to get out of their now abnormal blood sugar. (Milam)

Ross also says: "I have found the drug **tobacco** to be one of the fiercest and most complex addictors of all. Huge corporate financial resources have gone into making tobacco even more addictive, increasing both nicotine and sugar content of the formerly natural drug. Sweetness accounts for the majority of the cigarettes' additives. In deadliness, tobacco far exceeds heroin and cocaine."

She says that in order to overcome tobacco addiction once and for all, **most people will require some attention to metabolism**. Those who are thyroid imbalanced and try to do this with pills or patches, and without attention to thyroid, are not always doing themselves a favor.

The underlying metabolic situation that initially attracted users to the drug may still remain. In addition, the effect of the tobacco for such an extended time on the body, especially brain and nervous system, may make it imperative to then have some thyroid help for the recovery to be lasting. (Fukayama)

> **Many people who attempt to overcome tobacco addiction are thyroid imbalanced. Fixing the thyroid is crucial.**

If your metabolic balance is toward low thyroid, tobacco can be a stimulant. If your thyroid imbalance is toward high thyroid, tobacco could be a tranquilizer for you, making you feel calmer when you smoke. With this kind of pervasive problem, restoring proper thyroid function is vital if you wish to quit tobacco and stay off it.

In his book *UltraMetabolism*, Dr. Mark Hyman is very clear that thyroid needs to be utilized in these addiction situations. Many of his patients showed great benefit from thyroid hormone treatment. (Hyman) He recommends this approach for those who show any abnormal results on the same expanded thyroid panel we use, which includes TSH, Free T4 and Free T3, and thyroid antibodies (anti-TPO and anti-thyroglobulin). Sometimes he uses TRH stimulation tests, and even at times the 24-hour urine test for T3, which he feels can be helpful in hard-to-diagnose cases.

Once that diagnosis is made, he prefers to use a gradually increasing level of thyroid hormone. He also feels that there are times when the only way to determine if thyroid therapy will be of benefit is to actually *try* it. He recommends a trial for 2 to 3 months for these individuals.

William Jefferies, MD, is another endocrinologist convinced of the need for attention to thyroid, and sometimes adrenal, correction in people with addictions. Dr. Jefferies, a professor of endocrinology who has studied this area for decades, is certain that *cigarette smoking* and *coffee drinking* are significantly *related to the metabolism of thyroid and adrenal hormones.*

Dr. Jefferies recommends the concomitant use of cortisone and thyroid in recovery work. He feels that many people going through withdrawal may have need for extra cortisone and thyroid, having used up a lot of their own in prior chemical experiences. (Jefferies)

What This Science Really Means for You

It should be obvious by this point that one way to avoid some of these chemical traps that lead to eating disorders, substance abuse, and actual addiction is to **make sure that you are balanced in thyroid hormone**.

This means paying particular attention to symptoms, family history, associated illnesses, and physical signs, as well as looking closely at thyroid tests, to diagnose this issue accurately.

Addictions can arise insidiously, without warning. For example, imagine that you injured yourself enough to require a pain reliever. If you have thyroid issues, your pain pills might more easily become addicting.

A tranquilizer or sleep medicine required temporarily might soon become an actual master, rather than servant. With such common risks around us, why would anyone put up with an abnormal thyroid's altered brain chemistry? This just increases your risk, making you an easy target for addiction. Check your thyroid to better prevent this from happening.

The other important area of discussion is *treatment*. You may already be painfully aware of an eating disorder, or your proximity to substance abuse. You may even know you are addicted to caffeine, alcohol, tobacco, or sugar. So, what can you do about it?

Frequently, people work hard to become free of the substance, then try to reclaim their normal lives. They go to work, take time with friends, play with kids, have dinner with their spouse, watch movies, and attend sports events. Yet, during all of this, they frequently feel less than fulfilled or joyful.

Instead, they **feel that something is missing**, and they are eventually drawn back into their addiction. This scenario is unfortunately repeated thousands of times each day.

What is often missing is the proper level of thyroid hormone to support and control brain function optimally. (Joffe)

You may be missing enough thyroid power to get the same enjoyment and charge out of regular life as you have received while being on drugs. With proper thyroid balance, you could meet life's daily challenges with better stamina and reserve.

A Powerful Thyroid Solution

For a great many people, regaining normal thyroid levels can be a huge improvement. If you are among the 1 out of 10 who are thyroid challenged, it can give you your old life back—it might even provide you with a whole new lease on life.

Why not check more closely for a possible, even mild, thyroid abnormality? Then you can treat with simple benign thyroid hormone. It is likely that many individuals facing an addiction process need this additional help.

We live in a society that is known to be thyroid deficient. But experiencing an addiction (bulimia, alcoholism, etc.) for a certain number of years could also contribute to the likelihood of thyroid imbalance.

Are we suggesting that every person who has any type of addiction should be treated for thyroid problems? No, of course not.

However, it might be *1 person out of 10 who does require this additional type of support.* That is a large number of people who have not been treated fully. Identifying that one person (could it be you?) means increased interest in thyroid screening. Abundant research now suggests a greater use of thyroid awareness in the treatment of addiction and recovery. A large number of the people who have become addicted have become so because of their thyroid imbalances.

More research would be useful, but there is currently enough data to suggest that this maneuver—which has been so successful at our clinic, at Julia Ross's clinic, and at a few similar clinics across the nation—could now become more common in addiction treatment.

The simple addition of greater thyroid awareness might help you, regardless of what kind of program you pursue. Whether it's a 12-step program or cognitive behavioral therapy, just consider that optimal thyroid balance might be an important part of your recovery.

What happened with Maria's recovery? When we left her, her life was falling apart. Her desire to purge was leading to enormous guilt, remorse, and self-blame. This, coupled with her deteriorating physical health, led her to seek medical attention.

Maria's Story, Part 2

Maria originally went to an eating disorder specialist, who proceeded with the standard therapeutic interventions for this serious and complex illness. The results were not successful.

As with many participants in such programs, there is an altered metabolic set point from this condition that does not become readjusted simply by abstinence and therapy. (Joffe) Many need better thyroid balancing.

Maria's treatment was not proceeding well. As part of the routine workup, her TSH was tested and found normal, so she was not receiving thyroid care. A friend insisted she come see us for additional ideas.

It was only after coming to our clinic and receiving a full panel of thyroid tests that her antibodies revealed Hashimoto's thyroiditis. Then things really began to improve for Maria. Unfortunately, thyroid antibody testing is not a part of the normal workup, though her example suggests that perhaps it should be.

Based on the presence of thyroid antibodies, and the strongly suggestive history of thyroid disorders in her family, Maria was then diagnosed as having true hypothyroidism. Treatment of this easily controlled condition was the beginning of a favorable turn for her.

Special Challenges

- **Some doctors don't believe that there is a thyroid connection underlying the onset of anorexia or bulimia.** Instead, they feel that whatever thyroid abnormalities show up are due to the *effect* of the illness on the patient's metabolism, not vice versa.

- Also, and very important, **many anorectics and bulimics unfortunately abuse thyroid medication in their attempts to keep their weight under control.** This is another factor standing in the way of early diagnosis; it muddies the clinical picture and biases the doctor.

- We also readily admit that **there are many psychological and social considerations** when dealing with these insidious conditions. Careful

screening and an atmosphere conducive to honesty are crucial ingredients in this process.

- The decision to treat an addiction, especially an eating disorder,
with thyroid hormone must be carefully considered and expertly
carried out. The timing is delicate, and the patient has generally an
erratic sensitivity to thyroid medicines.

Maria's Story, Part 3

When Maria was first treated with Synthroid brand of synthetic
levothyroxine, she had an unfavorable reaction. She developed a skin
rash, most likely from the *Acacia* component of the Synthroid tablet
fillers, as well as stomach distress, which is an unusual response for
the population in general but is often seen with the very delicate
gastrointestinal systems of bulimics.

Rather than abandon her therapy, other types of thyroid
medicine were tried, until she had a favorable and highly beneficial
response to compounded thyroxine, in hypoallergenic capsules. Now,
after many years of similar patient responses, the "cleaner"
nonexcipient compounded preparations are our first choice for
thyroid addiction therapy.

Once tolerated by her system, the thyroid hormone began to
normalize her metabolism in a way that she had not experienced for
many years. The multipronged interventions of her eating disorder
program were now beginning to work more effectively and with
greater speed. She improved steadily over the next months and got
her eating, weight, and whole life back in balance.

Best of all, Maria now felt at the top of her game—just in time for
those college interviews. She performed well and was offered several
desirable options from which to choose.

Now, years later, Maria has maintained her recovery. The only
medicine she takes is her ongoing daily dose of thyroid hormone,
which she still needs. She is a successful lawyer who not only has
made her father proud but also has been able to re-secure title to the
family property in Mexico, where she is considered a local hero.
Despite the many faces of thyroid, Maria has managed to reclaim her
life, and her health.

Our Treatment Recommendations

Having spent years focusing on this condition, we have been able to identify products and activities that can best help to improve the person readily. Here we share some of our discoveries, both natural and pharmaceutical.

Over-the-Counter Remedies

By far, the best natural remedy for thyroid-caused neediness is the herbal medicine **ashwaganda**. This is frequently prescribed and well utilized in other countries, though less known in the United States. It is an excellent adaptogen, meaning that it regulates the hormone receptor sites for improved function.

This particular adaptogen has also been shown to favorably influence the conversion of T4 thyroid hormone into the active form of T3. Since trouble with such conversion is the reason for many people's neediness, this particular herb can be a true blessing. Take 100 mg of the standardized root powder twice daily on an empty stomach.

To help the thyroid restore proper balance, take 1,000 mg each of enlivening **tyrosine**, soothing **taurine**, and blood sugar–stabilizing **glutamine**. You can take all of the above once before breakfast, again mid-morning, and once again in late afternoon. These three amino acids can be extremely restorative to a depleted system.

Prescription Medicine

By far, the best medical treatment for the Needy thyroid type is the gentle but effective **compounded thyroxine**. A compounding pharmacy (see www.pccarx.com to find a compounder near you) can fill the prescription from your practitioner for a version of T4 that is generally smoother and better tolerated by Needy people than any other thyroid approach.

Because these thyroid pills are made up just for you, at the orders of your doctor, the strength of each pill can be totally individualized to your needs at each given time. It doesn't matter that the smallest off-the-shelf thyroxine is a 25-mg tablet; a compounding pharmacist can make for you a 5- or 10-mcg capsule for milder initiation of treatment. This allows for the more sensitive, carefully controlled upward titration that so many Needy types seem to require.

We recommend starting at 10 mcg per day, taken once in the morning well before breakfast. If this is tolerated comfortably, after a week move up to 20 mcg per day. After another week, move up to 30 mcg per day.

Continue in this fashion until up to 50 mcg daily. Then remain at 50 mcg daily for a month to evaluate progress. If five pills a day seems a lot to take, and if you like the results at that amount, your pharmacy compounder can then put all 50 mcg into one capsule at your next prescription refill.

Suppose 50 mcg has been successful temporarily, but then the initial benefit begins to fade. This simply means that your body has equilibrated to that initial plateau dose and now wants an increase. Once it is clear that thyroid medicine is tolerated and is helpful, then you are ready to search for your optimal dose.

We describe it as a search, because the end point is not determined simply by a lab test result. Instead, you are looking for improvement in symptoms and feelings as well. Dosage increases above 50 mcg can still be made in increments of 10 mcg, but the timing is more flexible.

Many people at our clinic find that each increase feels good initially, perhaps for a week or two or three, then begins to fade. Take heart and realize that this is a common experience, indicating that your body is asking for a higher dose of medicine. If your initial benefits at this current dose have faded somewhat, then try an initial 10 mcg daily.

The newly increased dose often feels good for a longer amount of time, but it, too, can begin to fade. If T3 or T4 levels are not too high on blood tests, then another increase of 10 mcg per day is in order.

Ultimately, Needy types often require up to 1 mcg per pound of body weight. That becomes, for example, 150 mcg per day for a 150-pound person, although many people do not need this much. The careful approach of "starting low and tapering up slow" allows your system to accommodate gradually to the increase in metabolism. **It is not a process that should be rushed.**

Eventually, there will be a dose that gives benefit that does *not* fade away over the weeks. The benefit from this more optimal dose can continue for many weeks, months, or years. In other words, you will have reached your optimal thyroid medicine level.

Once this phase is achieved, many of our clients tell us they feel like their old selves; they are less needy, experience fewer cravings and urges, and have less desire for the previous substances or habits of choice.

If you have a number of the symptoms or associated illnesses, then you might want to do a trial of thyroid hormone, even if all of the tests we've mentioned are normal. This trial of thyroid hormone should be administered carefully, with good guidance, starting at a very low dose and progressing upward gradually until a more normal dose for your body weight is reached, over a period of months.

If, in doing this, there is noticeable improvement in body or mental functions, mood, or cognitive ability, then you are indeed a candidate for longer-term use of thyroid hormone. The length of time to stay on thyroid medicine in such situations can be anywhere from several seasons of a year to several years.

Also, we want you to know how extremely helpful it has been for certain clinics to include thyroid treatment in their detoxification and recovery programs. Julia Ross of Recovery Systems credits the combination of over-the-counter and prescription thyroid remedies for a substantial part of her center's phenomenal success.

Finally, we once again recommend that if the above treatment maneuvers have not been helpful, or agreeable to your system, please consider trying different thyroid treatment, as presented in Chapters 4 through 7.

Although this chapter's regimen has been generally effective for the Needy person, some people with this mind-type might do better with another kind of thyroid treatment. In that case, your task is to find the thyroid protocol that works best for you. In addition, any thyroid treatment will work much better with the suggestions below.

Complementary Healing for Your Best Results

By Georjana Shames, LAc

Within this conception of the Five Elements and types of thyroid imbalance, we have seen how Moody, Edgy, Foggy, and Sleepy correspond to Fire (Heart Meridian), Wood (Liver Meridian), Earth (Spleen Meridian), and Water (Kidney Meridian). Now let us take a look at how the Needy type of person would correlate to the Metal Element (Lung Meridian).

The Lung Meridian is responsible for aspects of *respiration* (just as in allopathic medicine); yet, interestingly, in Chinese Medicine the **Lung**

Meridian corresponds to the **emotions of prolonged sadness and worry** (also known as grief).

What is it about prolonged symptoms of sadness or worry that can lead a Lung Meridian type of person to become susceptible to addictions, eating disorders, or obsessive drinking?

The answer lies in *how we cope* with sadness, depression, anxiety, or worry. When we experience these for prolonged periods, if we have not cultivated healthy ways of processing the emotional content of our lives, we will find unhealthy ways to navigate through the situation. They seem to work for a while, but these methods do not result in a lasting kind of peace.

For example, the Edgy type of person tries to cope with anxiety-provoking situations with irritation or full-blown rage, and that becomes the impetus for changing an uncomfortable situation. Though this temporarily satiates the person's desire to compensate for the uncertainty of his or her circumstances, it presents new problems.

No one really wants to go through life blinded by rage. It is very uncomfortable to walk around in a constant state of irritated dissatisfaction, as a Liver Meridian type of person will do if constantly out of balance.

The Lung Meridian type of person becomes Needy or addicted because his or her coping mechanism for prolonged sadness and worry (often caused by low thyroid) is to attempt to medicate or moderate the self. Without inner peace, the Lung Meridian type in Chinese Medicine is particularly susceptible to **feeling cut off from spirituality**, cut off from the ultimate meaning of life.

Substance addictions and eating disorders are as much *escapism* as they are facets of obsessive thinking. Attempts to manage grief using drugs, alcohol, work, sex, starvation, or some other form of self-destruction stem from our **natural but futile desire to trade discomfort for temporary peace**.

In order to truly heal, it is necessary to cultivate a more lasting peace.

POINTS TO PUSH

- Begin by locating the tender spot on the thenar eminence of the palm (which is the muscle that bulges with thumb movement), midway across the distance from the base of the thumb to the inner wrist. This point (called Lung 10) soothes sadness and fear at a deep level. It clears Heat from the Heart Meridian for anxiety and nourishes the Lung Meridian for long-standing grief that has transformed to agitation and addiction.

- Locate the area directly in the middle of the sternum (breastbone) in the fourth intercostal space. If you have difficulty identifying the fourth intercostal space, simply note that this point is located at about nipple level when you are lying face up on a flat surface. Massage this point (Ren 17) to "unbind the chest" for anxiety and grief. Additionally, it is a great way to soothe yourself and return to a kind of calm during periods of stress.

RECIPES AND REMEDIES

To make a recipe for soothing worry and breaking the cycle of addictions/eating disorders, prepare a romaine salad garnished with 5 ounces of roasted pumpkin slices, 5 ounces of shredded chicken, and 1 ounce each of cooked kidney beans, garbanzo beans, and purple potatoes. Add a side dish of 2 ripe sliced persimmons and a beverage of plum tea (boil 5 dried plums for 5 minutes and drink the liquid). Persimmon and plums bring rebellious energy down, for a calming effect when anxiety starts to rise.

Exercises that necessitate getting out of the house and breaking the patterns of prolonged worry and sadness are especially helpful for Needy types. Hiking with a friend is a great example, or attending group dancing events where you can meet other people interested in cultivating true health and at the same time enjoy physical exertion.

LIFESTYLE LIFTS

Lifestyle plays a particular role for Lung Meridian Needy types. In addition to the acupressure points and diet/exercise, it is critical to find healthy outlets for anxiety and grief, and possibly consider some form of spiritual practice. This does not have to be religious. It could certainly be, but for some people rigid parameters of the religion they grew up with serve only to increase anxiety and do not comfort the spirit.

Of course, the thyroid balance is a critical piece, but also finding some way to nourish a creative or spiritual life can help anchor you from the emotional storm. Whether it is going to temple or church, enjoying the beauty of the wilderness, participating in meditation retreats, singing in a choir, taking dance lessons, painting, listening to classical music, or anything else that appeals to you in a healthy way, it will help you overcome the cycle of neediness and addictions.

For some people, it can be extremely helpful to engage in therapeutic endeavors, including crafts, dance, and even brief stints of therapy. In our office, for example, Karilee Shames has the advance preparation both in psychiatry and holistic nursing to provide a wide range of treatment options, including emotional release, energy healing, and visualization.

THE BOTTOM LINE

- **Bulimia nervosa** consists of binge eating followed by compensatory efforts to minimize weight gain. These can include self-induced vomiting or excessive use of laxatives.

- **Anorexia nervosa**, the other main eating disorder, is characterized by a refusal to maintain a minimally normal body weight, along with an intense fear of gaining weight.

- **Thyroid plays a major role** in regulating overall eating behavior. Many addictive and substance abuse issues are **thyroid related**.

- Thyroid-related **changes in neurotransmitters**, especially serotonin, are an underlying cause of eating disorders in many unlucky women.

- Eating disorders are only one kind of craving often related to thyroid imbalance. Others include alcohol or tobacco addictions, abuse of prescribed medications, and addiction to narcotic or hallucinogenic substances.

- In desperate attempts to feel better, Needy mind-types will often self-medicate with these substances to treat an underlying metabolic discomfort.

- Some people with sluggish metabolisms have a decreased ability to stimulate their own brain's pleasure center with ordinary life.

- Thyroid imbalance, being largely inherited, may help explain why addictions are **often inherited**.

- For some people to overcome tobacco addiction once and for all, they need to **pay more attention to metabolism**, especially their thyroid function. Often missing is the proper level of **thyroid hormone** to **support brain function** optimally.

- Natural products that can help include **ashwaganda** and amino acids **taurine, tyrosine, and glutamine**.

- Generally, the most successful type of thyroid treatment for Needy types is **compounded levothyroxine**.
- Many people do very well working with a **compounding pharmacy** that allows them dosage flexibility and avoidance of potential allergy-producing fillers.
- **Acupuncture and Chinese Medicine** can be of enormous help in the difficult recovery from eating disorders and addiction.

RECOMMENDED ACTION PLAN

- For over-the-counter help with thyroid-related harmful habits, start with the strong herbal medicine *Withania somnifora*, commonly called **ashwaganda**. Try two pills twice daily of Mentalin, for example, from Metagenics.
- Boost its effectiveness with an **amino acid and thyroid support** formula (such as Energenics, also from Metagenics).
- If this is not fully successful, *combine* it with **a trial of prescription compounded levothyroxine** (T4 thyroid hormone) from a qualified practitioner, sending your prescription to a compounding pharmacy (www.pccarx.com).

PART III

Maintain a Lasting Cure

Chapter 9 presents the many specific items you can take or do, that will help to boost your overall function for the rest of your life.

Finally, Chapter 10 describes sensible lifestyle choices that are easy to implement, yet are of enormous additional benefit.

We hope this information helps you to maintain continued good health and well-being for many years to come.

9

Enhance Your Thyroid Treatment

Add Vitamins, Minerals, Herbs, Acupuncture, and Oriental Medicine

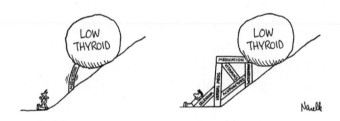

Have You Checked In with Your Inner Life Today?

Just as we believe in the power of the sciences, we also believe in the power of the arts. Both represent the highest forms of human expression and have evolved over centuries. One might ask, "Why do the arts often arise in the direst of places?" It appears that **art blooms in a space of need**. Amazingly, from the depths of our despair arise our truest gifts.

We have seen that each person, listening carefully to his or her life, can become a part of the next wave of consciousness in the ever-moving sea of human understanding. Taking the steps you need to take can serve as inspiration for many others around you. Remember, a butterfly flaps its wings and change happens across the globe.

As modern life has made abundantly clear, change happens. Structures and health can collapse, yet deep from the human spirit can arise positive visions, planted in times of need, caringly nurtured to fruition. What might look like illness and obstacles can really be opportunities if we just listen.

We can each be a part of that change opportunity.

New visions arise from within, as we sit in silence, listening to our breathing and to the steady beating of our own true heart. In silence, dreams can be revealed. It is an amazingly healing art form to then simply record the present of that moment of peace by keeping a journal.

Relieving stress is a great way to keep hormones comfortably flowing. For humans, that flow can also be nourished by dance, exercise, and massage. Preferably all. Laughter is great medicine, too!

We have shared information about what the thyroid does, what we believe is contributing to today's thyroid epidemic, and how these situations can affect mental health. We have discussed specific plans for those facing challenges with mood, memory, sleep, and related disorders of thyroid mental health.

This chapter is mainly about *things you can take* to boost and ensure improved thyroid function. (Our next chapter shares *things you can do* to maximize your program for optimal well-being.) We offer these ideas so that you can set the stage for maintaining long-term success.

Basic Nutritional Support

There are many ways to boost the effectiveness of your thyroid medicines. In general:

Thyroid sufferers require additional vitamins and minerals, due to the inherent digestive and absorption problems related to the underlying thyroid hormone metabolic imbalance.

We have already given you some suggestions to get you started:

1. You should already be taking the four supplements outlined in the **"Jump Start for All Mind-Types"** on page 66 of Chapter 3, in Part I.

2. In addition, you should also be taking the specific remedies recommended for your particular thyroid mind-type, as outlined in the appropriate chapter of Part II (Chapters 4 through 8).

3. The recommendations offered to you here in Part III are for boosting your health to that next level of long-term maintenance.

Optimal Additions to Further Enhance Your Program

We encourage you to experiment further by adding to your daily regimen certain simple items that will help you refine your program. Following are a variety of suggestions, often with the details listed in the Appendix and on our website, that can be of great benefit to you for maintaining a sense of comfort and ease for the long haul.

While you, like many thyroid sufferers, may always be a bit more sensitive in your own body, knowing about the supports below can allow you to live more fully and enjoy more of your life, while occasionally indulging in things that are pleasurable but not always healthy. Our goal is to help you to live a life that is full and balanced, without severe or unnecessary restrictions.

Mineral Support

- All too often quality minerals are neglected in metabolic balance. The general advice to take **an extra 500 mg of calcium** for bones, and an extra 20 mg ferrous fumerate **iron** if anemic, makes extremely good sense for people working with thyroid imbalance. *Note:* Take your **calcium and/or iron at a distinctly different time than thyroid hormone medicine**, preferably more than 4 hours

away from any thyroid dose. These particular minerals can interfere with absorption of thyroid hormone nutrients in your treatment plan.

- The most important mineral for a thyroid person, perhaps to many
readers' surprise, is *not* iodine. Instead, **selenium** is crucial for
those with thyroid challenges. "Selenium-dependent" enzymes
convert storage transport T4 thyroid into the active thyroid hormone T3. The enzyme is called 5-prime-deiodinase, a selenium-
dependent system of enzymes that is often not functioning properly
due to low selenium levels. We recommend **200 mcg daily** above
whatever is in your multivitamin.

- Another helpful item is **magnesium, 400 mg daily**, which can help
with many bodily aspects, including bowel function. If you take too
much, you may have loose stools, so then just cut back a bit.

Blood Sugar Regulation

Also quite important is **chromium at 200 mcg per day** above whatever is
in your multivitamin. Chromium is intimately involved with blood sugar
regulation, a process that many thyroid sufferers experience. Also, as mentioned below in the enzyme section, Formula 21: Sugar Digest (from
Enzymes, Inc.) can be extremely useful.

Beyond the Basics

In addition to the above important minerals, it is very useful to consider
oral *enzymes* as part of your thyroid program. Digestive enzymes are particularly appropriate, since thyroid abnormalities frequently result in the
process of digestion proceeding at too slow a rate. Adding digestive enzymes
to help an organ whose job is to convert food into energy makes good sense
for most people. For some thyroid sufferers it is essential.

Excellent Enzyme Support

A new company we are working with, called Enzymes, Inc., has created a
number of products specifically to help people with their thyroid-related

digestive disorders. One product Karilee has found amazingly helpful has been their **Formula 21: Sugar Digest**.

Her extreme sensitivity to sugars has for years made it difficult for her to eat a number of otherwise healthy and recommended food items, or even to have the occasional glass of wine, without feeling terrible afterward. Now, she simply takes two Sugar Digest capsules with a glass of wine or occasional semisweet food and is much more able to tolerate it.

- For those who feel worse after eating starch, Enzymes, Inc., also has **Formula 2: Starch Digest**.
- They also have **Formula 18: Fat Digest**.
- **Formula 601** is for **Gastric Comfort**.
- Their **Formula 12** is to help those needing to **Detox**.
- **Formula 801** helps with **Flora Balance**.
- If you are one of the millions who cannot digest dairy comfortably, you can either stop eating it, or use their **Formula 8** (lactase with probiotic support).

Additional Thyroid Boosting

- **Licorice** is considered an adaptogenic herb, meaning it can have a favorable regulatory effect on thyroid hormone binding sites. It also has been shown in medical center studies to help in the conversion of inactive T4 thyroid into the active hormone T3. An exceptionally effective version of this herbal medicine is available in Licorice Plus by Metagenics.
- Enzymes, Inc., also has a formula called **Thyroid Support**, specifically to help with thyroid boosting, utilizing a variety of important co-factors for this purpose.

Autoimmune Support

Although many practitioners acknowledge the importance of treating the underlying autoimmune cause of thyroid imbalance, few actually attempt it. Autoimmunity is not simply a sluggish immune system that can be boosted with ordinary interventions. In some ways it is an already overactive immune system. In other ways it is more of a confused immune system. A special and sophisticated remedy is needed.

- A complex and sophisticated herbal mix that is very helpful for autoimmune thyroid sufferers is **Padma Basic**. It is a combination of more than 15 separate herbs that work together in a variety of useful ways. It is a successful prescription medicine in Europe, under another name, but in the United States it can be purchased over the counter from a company called EcoNugenics (see Resources). A good dose is two tablets twice daily.

We simply do not have good Western medicines for rebalancing thyroid autoimmunity. Generally, our immune system protects us, but when it overfunctions, allergies often result. When the system is seriously over-functioning and confused, autoimmunity can be the result. Medicinal mushroom products have a way of repairing that situation.

- The product **10 Mushroom Formula** by EcoNugenics, taken in two tablets twice daily, is one effective way to help normalize a confused immune system.
- An Enzymes, Inc., product, **Thyroid Support**, mixes adaptogenic herbs with enzymes and minerals, including selenium.
- Those suffering sex hormone challenges can find relief with **Formula 501: Hormone Balance**, also from Enzymes, Inc.
- And, for those facing impaired neurological function, Enzymes, Inc.'s **Formula 19: Neuro Support** can help.

What makes Enzymes, Inc.'s products unusual is that each is a specifically created mix of enzymes (protease, amylase, lipase, cellulase, and others) that help to break down food products, working in combination with herbal and often mineral blends.

Note: If any of these products are not comfortably tolerated by your digestive system, you can discontinue and take **ProSol's Gastro Calm** or Enzymes, Inc.'s **Formula 601: Gastric Comfort** until you can tolerate proteases once more. These are all made by Enzymes, Inc.

- Pregnant women can take the digesting enzyme products, not the rest.
- Children can take **Digest Chewables** and **Chewable Digestion**. See our Resources section or website for more specific recommendations on these products.

In addition to enzymes, our digestive tracts often work better with additional friendly bacteria, such as acidophilus.

- There are many good versions of these **probiotics**, especially the ones containing billions of live organisms per serving. They are available in the form of liquids, capsules, or powders, many requiring refrigeration. Added to the GI tract daily or twice daily before eating, they help our normal intestinal flora to do their digestive jobs properly. We recommend one capsule twice daily of **Lacidofil DF** by Xymogen or **Ultra Dophilus DF** from Metagenics.

Ongoing Musculoskeletal and Overall Body Support

A thyroid-imbalanced person frequently exhibits difficulties in the muscles and joints. The blood supply, especially to the joints, is often very low. A sluggish or overactive thyroid often causes problems in these areas. Many of our patients with thyroid challenges have aches and pains in muscles and joints with no particular reason except for the thyroid involvement.

For this situation there are total-body enzymes that can be quite useful. Naturally Vitamins, a company based in Phoenix, has several special items to help the various mind-types as presented in this book.

- **For ongoing support of the Sleepy types**, we suggest **Fibrozym**, good for overall tissue repair. Many people lose sleep because of bodily discomfort. Fibrozym is composed of plant-based enzymes that normalize inflammatory response and improve overall tissue health.
- **For ongoing support of the Foggy types**, we suggest **Rutozym**, which Dr. Rich Shames has been taking for years due to his family history of heart problems. Remember that after menopause, women are more likely to have heart attacks.

Today's standard American diet and poor lifestyle habits leave many people with high cholesterol and hypertension, as well as circulatory disorders. People with excessive body fat are more likely to develop heart disease and stroke, even with no other risk factors. Obesity increases the strain on the heart, contributing to coronary heart disease.

It can also make diabetes more likely to develop. **Thyroid imbalance makes all of this worse.**

- For ongoing support of the Edgy types, **Medizym** (also available in a vegetarian version called Medizym V) can be very helpful. Karilee uses this and *loves* the cream for those dreadful muscular aches and pains. Experimental and clinical studies show that the specific systemic enzymes contained in Medizym work preventively to help the body maintain healthy immune system activity, reduce inflammation levels, and support natural tissue repair.

Long-Term Help for Those with Depression or Irritability

- **Hep-Forte** (from Naturally Vitamins) is a formulation of amino acids, protein, B vitamins, antioxidants, and other nutritional factors that have been shown to be important in maintenance and support of normal liver (hepatic) function. A popular seller worldwide, Hep-Forte offers nutritional support for overall liver health, particularly in cases of alcoholism, hepatic dysfunction due to hepatotoxic drugs and liver poison, and specifically male and female hormonal imbalance due to hepatic dysfunction.
- **Stimulin, also from Naturally Vitamins**, is a new approach to enhance stamina and renew energy. It helps promote better circulation and improve overall vascular health, supporting healthy libido, another common challenge for many thyroid patients.
- **Formula 50** is the Naturally Vitamins original protein formula used for 50 years for support of hair and nails, often a discouraging problem for thyroid-challenged women. Formula 50 contains protein and vitamin B_6 to support healthy hair and strong, shiny nails. The unique blend of amino acids nourishes and replenishes nutrients commonly lacking in a woman's diet; deficiencies can cause brittle, splitting, peeling nails and thinning hair.
- **Histame** is specifically designed by Naturally Vitamins for those of us with food intolerance, which so many of our patients have. Food intolerance is an adverse reaction to foods rich in histamine.

Effects can range from common digestive system problems including abdominal pain and spasms, diarrhea, constipation, and flatulence to headaches and skin rash.

Iodine: A Special Quandary

Iodine merits another special mention. Some practitioners and lay websites recommend that people with thyroid concerns ingest iodine in what are generally considered to be high doses. We consider that advice possibly quite problematic for those with autoimmune thyroid challenges.

It is paramount for most people in developing countries, especially in the interior of the continents, to supplement iodine. Lack of iodine in their diets has resulted in widespread and devastating diseases, including mental retardation, birth defects, and goiters. This is a terrible problem for possibly a billion inhabitants of the planet.

Most industrialized countries, however, have for generations provided iodine to their citizens in the form of iodized salt and iodinated bread dough conditioner. Iodine deficiency is much less of a risk for these individuals. In more recent times, however, bromine has replaced iodine in bread dough, and iodized salt has become less popular. Now scientists can observe mild resurfacing of these iodine problems in developed areas, including the United States.

The challenge is that iodine is a double-edged sword. For some people in industrialized countries, ingesting too much iodine makes autoimmune conditions worse. Too much iodinated thyroglobulin is a trigger for autoimmunity to exacerbate, often with devastating consequences for thyroid sufferers.

Our best recommendation is this: if you live near a coast, if you eat seafood, including sushi, or if you include sea vegetables (kelp, dulse, arame, hijiki) in your soups or salads, you are likely to be getting sufficient iodine and may not want to supplement separately, except under the direction of a good practitioner.

On the other hand, if you live inland—especially near the Great Lakes region of the US, where iodine is traditionally quite low—or if you are a person who has not used iodized salt on a regular basis and are living inland, and you also do not eat fish or ocean products, you could, in fact, be iodine deficient. Iodine is included in small amounts in many multivitamins.

People with definite autoimmune thyroid may wish to try to avoid excess iodine when possible. Those living in inland areas who don't eat fish or ocean vegetables may seek out iodized salt or the iodinated multivitamins.

The advice that everyone should have large amounts of iodine is something we cannot recommend.

Here is one reason we are cautious. In May 2003 the journal *Thyroid* published a study of schoolchildren in northwestern Greece. This area had been evaluated and designated as "thyroid insufficient" years ago. Public health efforts to improve that situation took the form of iodine prophylaxis, a method of ensuring that people in the communities take in extra iodine.

Years later the same population was once again evaluated. Results showed that the iodine deficiency had indeed been eliminated. But in its place was *a threefold increase in the prevalence of autoimmune thyroiditis* among the schoolchildren. Obviously this was not the desired outcome of such good intentions, yet it was not that surprising. Other studies had shown similar results. (Zois)

Here is another reason for our caution. An April 2009 report in the "Head and Neck Surgery" section of eMedicine online highlighted a study confirming earlier fears. Eric Lentsch, MD, and his colleagues at South Carolina College of Medicine showed that **papillary thyroid cancer** can be induced in animals with the administration of **excess iodine**. (Lentsch)

All in all, it seems that iodine is vitally important, but hundreds of studies attest to the notion that it needs to be approached with caution.

Iodine testing has improved in the last several years. For those who do wish to perform the new and potentially much more accurate kind of iodine testing, you may log on to www.CanaryClub.org to self-order special home test kits from Labrix Clinical Laboratory.

However, we want to be sure you understand that **to do the above test for your iodine levels, you need to ingest a significant amount of iodine in the form of pills that come with the kit.** We have been assured, by both doctors and researchers, that the kind of iodine used for these tests does not irritate preexistent autoimmunity problems. Still, we err on the side of caution when it comes to preventing harm to our patients. Exercise caution.

Boost Thyroid by Balancing Other Hormones

All of our discussions in this and previous chapters have related to a thyroid-challenged individual. In these people, thyroid imbalance is the main hormonal event, the center of attention, like the center ring of a three-ring circus.

Many people challenged by psychological symptoms have thyroid as their main hormonal problem.

In people for whom *thyroid is the main event*, related hormone systems may also need attention. Frequently, adrenal and sex gland rebalancing can be useful for **improving thyroid function**. Our additional suggestions below serve that purpose.

In our previous book *Feeling Fat, Fuzzy, or Frazzled?* we did more than mention these other two rings; we explored all three individually in some detail. This book is different.

What we are describing in this book are people who are definitely the thyroid endocrine-types.

Here, **whatever adrenal and sex hormone rebalancing we recommend is done in the context of improving thyroid status.** If you feel that either adrenal or reproductive issues might be your *main* factor, we refer you to www.FeelingFFF.com to do some of that foundational balancing first.

Sex Hormone Attention for Better Thyroid Function

It may help your thyroid system to rebalance your reproductive system using estrogen, progesterone, or testosterone, plus over-the-counter boosters of these hormones. This rebalancing of sex hormones can be a big help in optimizing overall thyroid function. We do not recommend taking strong doses of estrogen for this purpose. But when it is absolutely needed, small doses can help boost thyroid function in specific cases.

It is actually **progesterone**, rather than estrogen, that is generally most helpful for boosting and improving thyroid function. The use of testosterone can also be thyroid enhancing; if low in men or women, it can result in worse thyroid function.

We are not suggesting you just begin to take pills or start to slather hormone creams onto your skin. Instead:

> We recommend that you obtain *high-quality testing* on *thyroid, adrenal, and sex gland status* for a complete picture of which glands are malfunctioning *before initiating any treatment.*

If you do not have a doctor who will be open to your input in seeking high-quality hormone testing, or if you prefer the ease of home saliva testing, we suggest you go to www.CanaryClub.org and order your own home test kit. These are sent to you in the mail, allowing you to collect samples in the comfort of your home.

For those who have practitioners to work with who are knowledgeable in prescribing bioidentical hormones and saliva testing, you are in good hands. Many chiropractors, osteopathic or alternative practitioners, nurse practitioners, and women's health specialists have been using these methods to help balance hormones for years. The majority of obstetricians, gynecologists, and more traditional doctors are not yet aware of the increased accuracy of the home test option.

If you do not have a client-centered bioidentical hormone practitioner:

> You can still order your own kit, return your samples, obtain your results, and sign up with Dr. Rich Shames for a telephone coaching session.

During this initial 1-hour appointment (follow-ups are $^1/_2$ hour), he will review your lab results, take a comprehensive family history, and spend ample time explaining to you what your tests suggest and the beginning steps you need to take to help you feel better now. Follow-up appointments allow for polishing and fine-tuning your personalized program.

Adrenal Boosting for Better Thyroid Function

There is a whole other way to boost overall thyroid function, and that is to optimize adrenal performance. Frequently, adrenal function is low because the stress and pace of modern life have exhausted your supply of the main stress hormone, cortisol. Also, the same pollution affecting our thyroid glands is also impacting our adrenals, as they are both exquisitely sensitive tissues.

In our work, we have found that enhancing adrenal performance can be very useful in regaining thyroid balance. Items employed to do this, some of which were mentioned in earlier chapters, include:

- Certain vitamins, such as B_5 and B_6
- Selected herbal items, such as the adaptogens ginseng and rhodiola
- Glandular extracts from the adrenals of animals
- Over-the-counter pro-hormones like DHEA and pregnenolone
- Actual prescription hormones, such as bioidentical cortisol (hydrocortisone), used in very small doses

For proper use and dosage of any item above, please refer to our previous book, *Feeling Fat, Fuzzy or Frazzled*? The discussion there was mainly for the well-known adrenal involvement in anxiety. Still, you may also utilize adrenal interventions, if needed, to further rebalance thyroid-related difficulties concerning depression, memory, sleep, and neediness. Your Canary Club testing will reveal if adrenal involvement is significant for you.

Complementary Healing for Your Best Results

By Georjana Shames, LAc

Two millennia have passed since our fundamental Acupuncture text (called *The Yellow Emperor's Inner Classic*) was painstakingly etched into bamboo parchment, but the principles of diagnosis and treatment explicated in our ancient texts hold the same clinical significance today as they did thousands of years ago.

Acupuncture can be of special benefit amid our frenetic modern lifestyle, so often out of balance. Many people have regained their lost composure with the principles of the ancient Chinese way.

In this book, we have discussed how your thyroid health can benefit from massaging specific points on yourself to affect the energetic pathways for mental clarity and physical stamina. We have offered dietetic suggestions for improved gland function, which also help reduce emotional stress.

Now let's talk about how **actually *receiving* acupuncture from a practitioner can further boost your benefit**. A trained professional can insert stainless steel needles as thin as a strand of human hair into the skin points previously mentioned. This stimulates the points with more effectiveness than can be obtained with just finger pressure alone.

Generally 8 to 12 points are needled per treatment. These treatments are essentially painless, but they can occasionally cause a sense of tingling or fullness where the needles are placed, as the energy gathers. Almost always, the treatments are restful and surprisingly relaxing.

In Chinese Medicine, the basis of life for all beings is Qi (pronounced "chee"). Qi is the energy of our beating heart, the movement of our blood pulsing against arterial walls, our ability to breathe and stretch our legs and take off running.

Qi is the catalyst of both form and function. Each person's Qi creates the basis for her/his health and longevity.

When we employ needling techniques and herbal formulas, we instill a rebalancing of the patients' Qi from within, to restore equilibrium to the two interconnecting and mutually dependent forces of Yin and Yang. This guides the innate intelligence of the human body to nourish the meridians and internal organ systems, resulting in natural revitalization, with a recovery from disease.

Because acupuncture awakens the body's original intelligence to heal itself, it can benefit patients suffering from a vast spectrum of ailments—whether caused by bacteria in 200 BC, viruses in AD 2010, or internal factors such as a highly stressful lifestyle.

In our modern world, high stress and increasing pressures have become daily constants in almost everyone's life. We struggle to get out of bed, rush to drive in traffic, work long hours to prove our merit, become tired and wired from too much coffee and too little sleep, feel crushed under deadlines, scramble home to get dinner ready in time, argue over how to pay off new bills and old debt, mediate family difficulties, then try to finish the dishes and pack lunches and fold laundry and answer e-mails.

In Chinese Medicine, a fast-paced life with too much pressure without enough rest and rejuvenation is a leading cause of disease.

Living under stressful conditions day in and day out depletes the Qi and damages the Yin-Yang balance.

Fortunately, the human body is a remarkably resilient system, with an unparalleled ability to regain equilibrium. The Qi, Blood, Yin, and Yang can often be completely restored if one receives acupuncture, cultivating an approach to life that is focused on peace, happiness, moderation, and a healthy balance of work and relaxation.

In addition to using needles and herbs, most successful acupuncturists also share Acupuncture philosophy with their patients, including guidance for leading a balanced and sustainable life.

If you were able to see me for acupuncture in my San Francisco–area offices, I believe I could help you improve your situation. I am an oriental medicine thyroid specialist, who has also received acupuncture for years for my own thyroid condition. Doing so has benefited me immensely, more than words can express.

You are welcome to enjoy the video that explains more about my personal story of acupuncture for thyroid and how it can benefit your health at www.ThyroidAcupuncture.com. You can also browse testimonials from my patients here.

Finally, for those who live far from our offices and want an appointment with a local practitioner, here are some resources to assist you in finding a qualified acupuncturist in your area, so that you can receive the enormous benefit of treatments from a well-trained professional:

www.Acufinder.com
www.Acupuncturists.healthprofs.com/cam

On these sites, you can search by city or ZIP code, locating profiles of local acupuncturists in your area, with information about their specializations and their techniques. Some have videos you can watch; others offer free initial consultations by phone or in person.

THE BOTTOM LINE

- **Relieving internal stress** is a great way to keep hormones flowing.
- We recommend dance, exercise, massage, and laughter.
- Thyroid sufferers require **additional vitamins and minerals**, due to inherent digestive and absorption problems of thyroid malfunction.
- Keep an **open mind**. Any thyroid-balancing program can be further improved with additional supportive vitamins and minerals, herbal medicines, appropriate enzymes, attention to the underlying autoimmune issue, and focus on related medical/hormonal concerns.

RECOMMENDED ACTION PLAN

- You should already be taking supplements as outlined in the **"Jump Start for All Mind-Types"** (Chapter 3).
- You should also be taking the **"Specific Remedies"** recommended for **your particular thyroid mind-type**, as outlined in the appropriate chapter of Part II (Chapters 4 through 8).
- Follow this Long-Term Maintenance Program:

  — Take an extra 500 mg **calcium** for bones, and extra 20 mg ferrous fumerate **iron** if anemic, 4 hours before or after thyroid hormone.

  — Add 200 mcg **selenium** daily for improved thyroid function.

  — Add **magnesium**, 400 mg daily, to help with bowel flow.

  — For blood sugar regulation, add **chromium** at 200 mcg daily.

  — Add **digestive enzymes** to help convert food into energy.

  — Take the herbal supplement **licorice** to help conversion of T4 into active T3.

  — Include **Padma Basic** for better immune system function.

  — **Probiotics** can help with better digestion and assimilation.

  — Enhance your self-care with **digestive and systemic enzymes**, trying them *one at a time* so you can evaluate results.

  — Balance adrenal and sex hormones to boost thyroid function.

  — Remember to **test your hormones** *before* trying to fix them.

  — In Chinese Medicine, a **fast-paced life** with too much pressure and **not enough rejuvenation** is a leading cause of disease.

  — Consider the benefits of **acupuncture for faster results** that will be longer lasting.

- Make your long-term maintenance personal and individualized using the many options offered above.
- Extra iodine is sometimes useful, but sometimes best avoided.
- Choose items that feel consistent with your wallet, beliefs, and interests.

10

Enjoy a More Powerful Lifestyle

Making Time for Nutrition, Stress Reduction, Exercise, Bodywork, and Spirituality

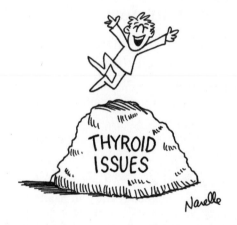

Narelle

Most machines come with an instruction manual that specifies that *maintenance is required*. Unfortunately, we do not come with user manuals.

You will forge your own path to better health, but in order to help guide you on your journey, we include little pearls that we hope you will take to heart—if not now, then perhaps at another time.

It is our prayer that this book does more than educate you about its specific topic. We also want you to feel more whole, coming away with a variety of little gems that eventually help to light up your life. That is our commitment, and our prayer. Your empowerment, and reclaiming of your full health, is our reward ... and a lovely reward it is. Our ideas for supporting your empowerment continue to evolve around the critical *central value of self-care* in working your way through today's "modern medical machine."

Informed health consumers can organize and activate, each becoming his or her own best health advocate, together working toward better health options.

Especially in the field of mental health, where it is increasingly more difficult to access optimal care, family involvement is crucial. With most mental health units that used to care for our relatives and friends now dismantled, what options remain?

There may be a much better option. When you first notice odd behavioral symptoms, fix the thyroid!

Good News for Health Consumers

Today more than ever, health consumers are directing their own care, using their minds and voices to access options more consistent with their own beliefs and values. Despite the many dictates of modern medicine, when it comes down to health care, you must speak out on your own behalf, or for those you love.

Health care is simply another form of big business. The same laws of finance operate as with any business.

You have a right to choose what you pay for, and to decide what should happen, *especially* when it comes to your body and your health.

Even if you, like millions today, have hit upon hard financial times, you still deserve to be adequately cared for, within the constraints of the current system. Human dignities must be honored while caring for sick people, whether physically or mentally ill.

We highly recommend that you:

- Educate yourself.
- Demand better health care.
- Inform your practitioners and seek their support.
- Seek practitioners who will work with you on your goals.
- Join consumer advocacy groups for greater power.

Rather than just continuing to fix the devastating end results of poor thyroid care, we prefer a more proactive approach that teaches people to care for themselves, so they can approach health options in a balanced, assertive manner. **Not only is it your choice, it is also *your responsibility* to make the best decisions for your own life and health.**

Today, we must all learn to claim our own power, to become our own ultimate decision maker, and to help tame the thrashing medical monster, if only by grabbing its tail and holding on for dear life until a better system is put in place.

> **With greater mental focus and knowledge, a stronger sense of well-being, and a clear sense of how to proceed, we can begin to heal ourselves.**

Building a New Era in Health Care

Together, in small local groups or online, we can build health communities that can make a difference. Sharing our knowledge and support, we can become beacons of light for our next generation's medical care. We can now take what we have learned and run with it.

We can share stories from medicine's history, the women's and men's movements, and our family. We can all learn to sing out together for greater healthy change.

Speaking out your concerns in small group settings can be the first step toward our collective advancement. Individuals can sharpen skills in these groups, allowing those with clear passion and purpose to rise to leadership, or to rotate leadership, according to how your group chooses to form itself.

Ultimately, leaders from within groups can join forces in cyber-groups, phone conferencing, or eventually leading seminars. These groups will meditate and continue to affirm positive visions, so that leaders can emerge and speak out for our world, making it better with our voices joined.

> **Healing is a process, not a state of being. We are constantly evolving as humans, as teachers, as leaders. Forgiveness is the fastest route through any situation. Waiting is the mark of someone who doubts. Action is the mark of someone who leads. Be the change you seek.**

Be sure to see the Appendix at the back of this book for information about finding or creating groups, and locating good local practitioners.

Embracing Lifestyle Changes

Thyroid treatment alone, even when boosted with ideas suggested in Chapter 9, is sometimes not as effective as one might like. For some people, old habits—like overeating, smoking, or dependence on alcohol—can easily undermine healing. For others, unmanaged stress is the culprit.

In our fast-paced lives, many people seem to thrive on pushing the edges, moving quickly and accomplishing much, and taking great pride in their accomplishments. In the long haul, this tendency can be harmful. While we *can* sometimes do it all, it is not always in our best interest to do so.

Now it is time to synthesize our evolving knowledge. Every person can get involved on some level, so you are not only helping yourself, but helping others facing similar issues. Healing lifestyle choices are generally broken down into the following categories:

- Sensible nutrition
- Stress reduction
- Enjoyable exercise
- Rejuvenating bodywork
- Spiritual growth

Each of these will be explored separately in the discussion below, but first allow us to describe the fundamental basis for these categories.

We once again mention that to heal superbly well, you may want to join or create your own thyroid support group, where you can meet and share with others facing thyroid-induced mental health challenges. You might find yourself discussing which treatments work well and which do not.

Soon, consumers will be helping practitioners to find new pathways to health. While tempting, it does not seem to help much to blame doctors, many of whom may not have been well educated in subtle thyroid issues or the so-called alternative methods of working with disease. For a variety of reasons, many of our patients are also finding their experiences with endocrinologists frustrating.

Instead, we can learn together, uncovering the special mysteries of having these chronic conditions and, ultimately, informing our caregivers. If your physician is too busy, or not interested, it's best to move on. Find someone who is open-minded and will listen to your ideas without demeaning you for wanting a more comprehensive view.

We feel fortunate to have learned so much about this new healing from our clients. We have incorporated this information and taken new directions, in the hopes that it would improve our practice, while helping you to heal more fully. We thank you all for sharing your honesty.

For those who send us correspondence, we only hope you realize how much your stories have meant to us, even when we have not been able to respond personally. You have informed our work, allowing us to share more deeply.

Together, we can advance this important new field of psychoneuroendocrinology. Let us begin with simple ideas to round out your plan.

Commonsense Wisdom for Healing Our Lives

These suggestions come from the foundation of the integrative health movement we became involved with decades ago. After our medical training came this additional understanding about the soul of medicine.

We offer deep gratitude to all those who have walked this sometimes rocky course with us, since the beginning of the US movement nearly 40 years ago. There have been medical visionaries, such as Norm Shealy, Gladys McGarey, Andrew Weil, Larry Dossey, and many others, still walking on this unfolding path to design new and better forms of medicine.

Here are our thoughts on why this is especially important to address now.

- Modern medicine is unsustainable without modifications.
- People are suffering enormously due to the lucrative excesses of pharmacology, surgery, and radiation that overwhelm our bodies' ability to restore their own health.
- Each of these treatments may be helpful in certain specific situations. **Applying them too generally can be harmful** to us.
- Although isolated small symptoms can be treated one by one, we can encounter serious excesses if we have a long list of significant symptoms, each requiring treatment. For better solutions, modern **medicine can look to a more integrative approach**, treating the whole person, using tools from ancient and modern practice.

"Thyroid Recovery"— Our Shared Goal

In this chapter, we recommend that you become *proactive*, and insist on more effective medicines, supplements, or activities, when appropriate. Use them in various combinations as needed, until you actually reach your true endpoint, which is *full recovery.*

It is of crucial importance to reach and maintain truly optimal thyroid status in order to meet your full life potential. Far too often, the upward titration of thyroid medication is *stopped prematurely* based on one overrated blood test result, rather than looking at the whole person and his or her array of only partially resolved symptoms.

Likewise, booster supplements and integrative therapies are commonly reduced before full thyroid recovery has been attained. Most often this is a result of the person feeling better, yet not realizing how much better he or she could actually become.

A key component of this success is to realize this critical key point:

> **Thyroid treatment, whether natural or by prescription, is often not nearly as effective as thyroid treatment combined with targeted lifestyle enhancements.**

When you begin to add lifestyle changes to the details of this program, you may feel as Sleeping Beauty did awakening from her long sleep. And, we promise you—there will be beauty to behold!

"Full Recovery"—Reclaiming Your Whole Self

In general, full recovery means that you have unlocked a door that was previously accessible to you, even if only as a child. You now rediscover that door. Amazingly, after all these years, you have finally found the key to opening it.

Inside, you encounter treasures that have collected dust, having for so long remained untouched. They have never been fully forgotten. In fact, in younger years, you may have yearned for these aspects, as they gradually began to fade from your life.

Recently, these parts of your life may have appeared more as dreams in some faraway aspects of your psyche, rather than as parts of you that still exist inside. But as they beckon, you will not only remember but also instantly embrace them.

> You can reclaim your childlike wonder, your sense of hopefulness, or even your long-forgotten laughter. They are like old friends that you instantly recognize and want to visit with again.

Now, you walk toward them and touch one forgotten part of your earlier life. It awakens, stretching, as if from a long slumber. The Rip Van Winkle aspects inside of you arise after years of disuse and begin to creak back into action. You do not feel different than you did as a younger person; you feel exactly as you did back then—more connected, more hopeful, more vital and alive.

> Full recovery for a person who has lost touch with these aspects can be the greatest gift you have ever received.

It can feel like a balm applied to soothe your aching soul, music to once-deaf ears, or a mother's loving touch. Once you feel it, you will recognize what you have given to yourself, the most alive *you* possible. You and your loved ones may well be delighted.

Now that you have made it this far, you have done the hard work; the steps yet to be taken are like icing on the cake. They will help you to feel even better, more alive, and more productive for the long haul.

So let's get started, first with nutrition, then with stress reduction, exercise, and bodywork, and ending with spiritual growth.

Sensible Nutrition

In addition to giving our car gas, we must also use special products to help maintain the vehicle. We need windshield washing fluids, brake fluids, quality oil that is regularly changed, spark plugs, lightbulbs that require changing, and many other aspects of care that help keep the car in good shape for a longer life.

So it is with our bodies. What we feed to our bodies must contain enough energy to make our bodies go, and to keep them going. If we pour sand into the gas tank, our car will not be going far. If we eat only greasy, fried, or sugared foods, we will likewise not be going far.

Our best sense, as integrative practitioners, is to **use the most natural food items available** without contributing to the pollution in our air and water. We suggest eating foods in their most natural form possible, and learning to eat them wisely so as to enhance the thyroid system.

Food is nourishment for our bodies. It is taken in, chewed, broken down by enzymes in the saliva and digestive tract, and the resulting nutrients carried throughout the bloodstream. The human body operates at much lower temperatures than chemical reactions in test tubes. Enzymes are catalysts that break down or assemble the chemicals of life, allowing these reactions to occur at a lower temperature and at the specific time and place needed.

Our digestive process allows us to break down foods into energy that we use and to eliminate those aspects not needed. Caring for our digestive tract is something we don't normally think about. Yet in people with sluggish digestion, there can be many resulting problems.

Eat pure, simple foods as often as possible. Fruits, vegetables, juices, grains, beans, and similar natural whole foods have been eaten to sustain humanity for thousands of years. Now we have reached a crisis point, where people are eating "entertainment" food that cannot honestly be considered proper food, as it is sorely lacking in nourishment. Entertainment foods include ice cream, candies, cookies, cake, chips, pizza, and other things that taste too good to be true.

> **People with lowered thyroid function often digest so slowly that toxic buildup occurs inside of them, making them feel unhealthy.**

When low thyroid results in poor digestion, giving the body the right amounts of thyroid hormone can be restorative on every level. Accumulation of toxic substances in our bodies can definitely impact the way we behave.

Surviving and Thriving in Today's World

In our fast-paced culture, many people find that they are stuck without decent nutrition, either on the road or in the workplace. Foods provided in institutional settings are often laden with chemicals that can make the food last longer and taste better, but leave us feeling worse.

People with sluggish metabolisms are frequently more sensitive to environmental toxins, including those in foods they ingest. Eating these chemicals can easily result in the person feeling dizzy, tired, or unable to think clearly—none of which helps our lives, or our mental health.

Nurses, as an example, today work 12-hour shifts in hospitals that do not feed them adequately. Doctors grab a cheese sandwich as they move from patient to patient throughout the days and nights. One even wonders whether the dieticians in some hospitals would ever choose to eat for themselves what they are supplying to sick people. As practitioners who have practiced outside of hospitals for years, we find this so odd. Surely by now the medical system has begun to recognize that in order to heal, people need exceptionally healthy foods? We are happy to say that more hospitals are seeing the senselessness of this mode of being and are revising their menus to include more organic and healthy foods.

Healing Foods

The USDA food recommendations have undergone revisions in recent years, as our understanding of vital foods has changed. People are beginning to recognize that we are only as healthy as the foods we ingest.

We start by suggesting you consider eating as much **organic food** as possible. Thyroid function is very sensitive to synthetic chemicals and appreciates when you minimize your exposure to these in food, air, and water. The fewer toxic substances you ingest, the less your liver has to work to overcome the burden of these substances. This means eating organic whenever possible, and choosing your restaurants and markets as carefully as you can.

For general purposes, we suggest that you keep away from fatty foods, fried foods, and heavy use of salt or spices. In other words, eat lightly and moderately.

We recommend a diet high in fiber and low in calories, featuring more vegetables and fruits, beans, seeds, and sprouts. High-fiber foods, including prunes and prune juice, keep the bowels moving. Having sufficient bowel movement is key. Slow bowels allow toxins to accumulate in the intestines, contributing to our feeling poor.

We also advise eating less meat and less dairy. This will help to lower autoimmunity, allowing you to feel better. Many of the chemicals that are best to avoid are concentrated in the *fat* of meats and dairy products. The less meat and dairy you eat, the less is your body's burden of these thyroid-hormone-disrupting toxins.

When you do eat meat, consider cutting your portion in half, eating smaller amounts at each meal. In addition, if you choose to grill, remember that the black charcoal's effects that make the food taste so good are contributing to cancers. Go easy on the grilling; stop before it's burned. As with so many situations, moderation is the key to a healthier life.

Karilee's very wise Gramma Fanny always said, "Too much of anything is no good."

Dairy is often tasty, but it upsets those with lactose intolerance. If you get gas, stomach cramps, constipation, or other uncomfortable symptoms after eating cheese or ice cream, adjust your diet accordingly and consider some of the enzymatic products listed in Chapter 9.

While ice cream may feel like an essential food to some of us, we can assure you it is not. You can take lactase tablets to help you digest when you do indulge; many are available now even in grocery stores. You can also browse health food stores and experiment with the great-tasting rice or soy "ice creams" that have much less fat and no dairy. Nut ice creams made without dairy are delicious.

Eat simply. You might try to find ways to purchase more of your food in bags you fill yourself from bulk bins, or shop at health food stores more often. There are a great many nonanimal protein sources, including avocado, olives, nuts, tofu (in small amounts), and others to sustain you.

Use good oils. There are "good fats," as opposed to the hydrogenated vegetable oils used in many processed foods we eat. We urge you to try to avoid these hydrogenated oils, as they interfere with metabolism.

Munch on nuts. For those with ups and downs related to sugar metabolism, eating a small handful of nuts every few hours will ensure adequate protein supply to balance out sugar. Chew carefully.

Read the labels on food packages. If you cannot pronounce all the ingredients, it may be advisable not to eat it. The chemicals used to preserve food can confuse the body's efforts to metabolize effectively. The popular diets of Drs. Pritikin, Ornish, and McDougall also make similar suggestions.

We do not recommend skipping breakfast. In fact, we suggest eating at regular intervals, even if it's only small healthy snacks. After a night's sleep, the body needs energy. For many thyroid patients, eating small meals throughout the day rather than large meals works best for metabolism.

Finally, we recommend steering clear of the CATS—caffeine, alcohol, tobacco, and sugar—which are metabolically problematic for thyroid types.

Coffee smells great and gives a punch to help you get through the day. Only problem is, however, what goes up must come down. Predictably, you will crash after coffee and require more coffee, sugar, or both, just to stay afloat. **Herbal teas give a nice lift without caffeine.**

Chocolate is something many of our patients adore. While it tastes delicious, it may not be your best friend. Chocolate has xanthines, which are like caffeine. Medical studies do not confirm true psychological benefit. (Golomb)

Alcohol should be considered a treat. Most of us realize that it must be broken down in the liver, which can at times add undue stress. Some are also sensitive to the added chemicals, such as **sulfites in wines**, which prevent them from spoiling. There are a few organic or "no sulfite added" brands of wine we know of in California, including Frey, Badger Mountain, and a few biodynamically grown brands to minimize toxic exposures.

Beer has additional yeast, something most of us could do without. For those plagued with excess *Candida albicans* (overgrowth of yeast after long exposure to antibiotics, birth control pills, or major sugar), yeasty beer is not a good choice. Those with sensitive digestion do not break it down or tolerate it well. Once in a while, on a hot Mexican beach, however, a beer is just what the doctor ordered (and enjoys!).

Do your best to use less and less sugar in your cooking. Eventually, your taste buds adapt to less, and you won't miss the excess sweet taste.

For those growing their own food, **use fewer chemical pesticides** and more natural pest controllers. (In our now small garden, which was larger when we had children, we have always used cayenne pepper mixed with water in a sprayer to help contain aphids and pests. The same holds true for household chemicals. Deborah Dadd has many excellent suggestions in her book *Home Safe Home*.)

Anything we can do to minimize our own toxic burden is our gift to ourselves. Anything we do to minimize our burden to the Earth is our gift to our grandchildren.

What to Avoid

Try to avoid using **NutraSweet and other artificial chemicals** that can scramble the body's metabolism. Most of our clinic patients feel a whole lot better just giving up artificial sweeteners.

There are a number of **goitrogens**—foods that adversely impact thyroid function. You need to cook them well and eat small amounts, or avoid them. One of the biggest is soy. Others include cruciferous vegetables like broccoli, cauliflower, and others from the Brassica family.

It may be tempting to use stimulants, even natural ones, but **we highly recommend against using either prescription or natural stimulants**. Herbs like ephedra, guarana, and gotu kola—in many of today's "energy" drinks—might seem to temporarily boost metabolism, but they are not helpful for the restoration of your depleted glands and organs.

Despite the fact that strong energy drinks line the exit shelves of most stores today, do not give in! Breathe deeply and fully, jump up and down, and exercise frequently during your day. You can restore your own energy for life in better ways that will ensure wellness for the long haul.

Cleaning and Cleansing

In daily life, **avoid heavy-duty cleaners**. Although they clean well, they give higher levels of exposure to chemicals that tax the immunity. Clean your house with products that are nontoxic whenever possible.

You can learn how to clean your house with vinegar, club soda, and other natural items, again avoiding the exposures that slow down or confuse thyroid function. Some chemicals have a label "caution," which is mild; "warning" is stronger; and if the label says "danger," this is likely to be a product you'd best avoid. Always use all-purpose products rather than extra-strength. Keep doors and windows open while cleaning to avoid overpowering smells.

Inside the house, be wary of using any toxic chemicals if you can possibly avoid them. (In our home, we have mixed peanut butter with boric acid to contain roaches. Now hardware stores sell noninsecticide "roach motels," where roaches can enter but not escape. We also found a chemical-free machine that traps mosquitoes.)

Now let us move on to **body care products**, which most of us use. Do your best to find skin creams that are not filled with toxic chemicals.

If you can't pronounce the ingredients, don't slather it on your skin.

Remember that our *skin* is our *largest organ for elimination*. Keep your pores open with regular hot showers and baths. In the European tradition, you can open them with heat, then close them with cold. Skin brushing can help to remove older "dead" cells, so that your skin can renew and rejuvenate. Olive oil is used the world over for healthier skin.

Our **teeth** can also be cleaned without ingesting chemicals. Health food stores have many low-synthetic, fluoride-free toothpaste options that are not so irritating to our immune systems. Some folks use sea salt; some rinse with peroxide occasionally. If your dentist insists on your having fluoride, best to do it in trays—be sure *not to swallow*. Many thyroid-compromised people elect to pass on the fluoride treatments for reasons already discussed.

In addition to minimizing your exposure to toxic chemicals, you may want to *engage in body-cleansing activities periodically*. These can include short fasts. Eating simple pure food such as only soup or salad, adding green fresh vegetable juices, and drinking lots of water for even 1 day each week can give the organs a rest and nourish your body.

Taking a week, or just 3 days, of eating nothing but pure simple foods (brown rice, cooked vegetables, lots of water between meals) can help to detoxify. If you do this and are feeling better after the third day, you may wish to continue for a longer time. We recommend doing this with the oversight of a competent practitioner.

For those who use sugar or alcohol regularly, keep in mind that it can take 3 full days for your body to cleanse and start feeling better. People who have been eating poorly can occasionally experience headaches while detoxifying, but after a while they tend to feel like a new person.

For those with juicers or very strong blenders like Vitamix, you can make a fresh cup of vegetable juice each morning.

This is truly a great way to start your day. Or mix veggies with water or nut milks in your Vitamix to begin your day right. Some people include high-quality whey protein powders in this drink. This type of daily green drink (with a small amount of carrot just to make it taste better) can help make the commonly acidic body slightly more alkaline, which helps in overall thyroid function.

More Self-Care Suggestions

- Use natural organic skin, hair, and body care products whenever possible.

- Many cultures use olive oil and cocoa butter for skin and hair.

- Avocado and papaya with a little honey make a delicious face mask.

- A saline nasal rinse can help those facing sinus problems.

- Scrubbing the skin with a loofah or skin brush can help remove debris and allow the skin to function more efficiently as a cleansing mechanism.

- Many folks take occasional coffee enemas to expel toxins. You can purchase disposable enema bags online, or use a hot water bottle with a long enema cord. Boil 3 tablespoons organic coffee in 2 cups purified water for 2 to 3 minutes; strain and cool to body temperature. It's best to do this on an empty stomach in the morning, while lying on your right side, curled up. Do not overfill. It is said that after you hold for 12 minutes, while breathing, caffeine opens the hepato-portal duct, allowing the liver to cleanse. Best to ingest alkaline products after this (such as greens) to balance acid. Some folks cleanse with hearty greens that have enzymes, like wheat grass. Follow with probiotics.

A Healthier Digestion Means Fewer Parasites

We know; you'd rather not talk about the topic of intestinal parasites. We feel the same way. But the reality is that in our fast-paced, germ-altered world, little creatures can really be just about anywhere—and that includes on our food. Moreover, altered inner flora can affect immune system balance. Most of our immunity (antibody-producing B cells) is in clumps called Peyer's patches, scattered throughout the intestine.

Wash your veggies, as many of us have learned to do, especially after the recent *E. coli* outbreaks. Little microscopic creatures may be as puzzled as the rest of us when it comes to trying to make sense of today's unpredictable world, complete with mutating germs. It's wild out there.

The best we can do is to retreat at times, and some of those healing times need to be devoted to the less-than-pleasant tasks that humans need to do for self-care, such as cleaning our bodies, cleaning our minds, cleaning our houses, cleaning our refrigerators.

Some people feel better after cleansing their intestines either by enema or colonic. Most would prefer not to talk about such distasteful ideas; it is not considered genteel.

But especially if you have traveled and spent time in Third World countries, checking for parasites is an important piece of today's modern life. The stress on our immune systems has eroded the ability of our internal defenses to do as great a job as previously of screening out organisms that do not belong.

If you have been losing weight or feeling tired, or have malaise or irritable bowel, then **along with your total thyroid evaluation, consider checking by stool test for parasites**. They're like bad neighbors that you sometimes have to deal with; if you're lucky, you can flush them out.

Eradicating Parasites of Any Kind

Lowering the parasitic load can be like taking a thorn out of the side of the immune system. Any person can eat food with microscopic creatures on it that can multiply inside. Leave no stone unturned on your path to wholeness. Seek out a qualified practitioner who can help you. Do the recommended stool tests, and find out what needs further help.

And, as a crucial aside, *if some of your parasites happen to be human,* you may need to remove them as well. Rather unfortunately for the rest of us, some people have learned to survive by sucking the life out of others, metaphysically speaking. Ultimately, we find that our best health comes from keeping them and their energies away from us.

Based on the discussions shared in earlier chapters, the odds are growing that in each of our lives, on a daily basis, we are encountering human parasites regularly. When you encounter one, you may find yourself feeling absolutely drained. You might feel depleted, low in energy, resentful, or otherwise generally unhappy. This can be a first clue that you need to review your relationships (and your intestines and your thyroid), and adjust them each accordingly. Keeping ourselves strong and healthy requires vigilant observation and daily care.

The Healing Miracle of Water

Water is the largest component of our bodies. Our bodily systems use water in countless ways: to make blood, flush toxins, digest food and break it down into energy for life, and maintain body temperature.

There is much debate today about the quality of our waters. Our oceans are dying; some rivers and streams are so polluted that fish cannot live in them. Yet somehow we must drink large amounts of water daily just to survive.

Many of us are buying up water in plastic bottles, hoping to remain healthier. However, in doing this we cannot keep contributing to the mountains of plastic debris that are accumulating. Recent reports are also informing us that the bottled waters are not regulated, and many brands may not be superior to what we are receiving out of our taps. (Keegan)

For all these reasons, it can be quite useful to use **water filters**. Extraneous chemicals that could be damaging thyroid function can be largely, if not totally, filtered out, giving your eliminative organs a needed rest. These can include heavy metals, bacteria, parasites, and algae.

Most superior filters can rid chlorine from drinking water, but only special ones using reverse osmosis or distillation can take out the fluoride. For those new to our recommendations, let's talk about fluoride. We cannot do the subject justice here, but we can share a few simple thoughts on our long-standing views expressed in our other books.

The Sad Controversial Case
of Fluoridated Water

Those who have read our previous books know that we are proud to be "fluoro-phobes." This is the intentionally disrespectful name given by industry to individual citizens who are rightfully wary of adding question-able waste product substances like hydrofluosilicic acid to our drinking water for greater corporate profit.

Surprise! It is not sodium fluoride that is added to our drinking water to make it fluoridated (even though the earliest city comparison studies were performed using sodium fluoride). It is an industrial waste product that is contaminated with lead and other toxins, causing children to lose IQ points in communities across the world (studied in China). Despite the vast resources of the American Dental Association, which appears to be doing the bidding of the phosphate fertilizer industries in unconsciously promoting this practice, we—like many good scientists—believe it is not safe in the long run. We consider it a misguided, outdated policy. As we have said in other books, to us it is "a bad idea whose time has passed."

If we as health professionals are not able to tell our truth to you, our trusted readers, then we end up ultimately questioning our own value and worth. We opt instead for taking the risk, telling you what we have learned as we understand it, rather than adopting any party line. We trust in your ability to sift through information and make your own best decisions.

Regarding fluoride, we hold these truths to be self-evident (and easily confirmed):

Sodium fluoride was in years past used in hospitals to slow down thyroid function for people with overactive thyroid.

Today much of what passes for "fluoride" added to our drinking water is actually hydrofluosilicic acid, an industrial waste product.

Even more insulting is its contamination with lead and other heavy metals. This magnifies the harmful effects of the fluoride, and perhaps most pertinent to this book, combined they can more easily affect thyroid, thereby detracting from mental function.

There are also those pesky "freedom of choice issues" inherent in add-ing *anything* to our public drinking waters, let alone something that has been **proven to slow down thyroid function** in millions of citizens. This little mistake, left over from the Cold War times, could now be affecting millions of people, some of whom are understandably wondering why there is such an epidemic of low thyroid these days.

> **We can learn to use food, clean water, and other lifestyle modifica-tions as our best defense against illness.**

Currently, there are inexpensive versions of carbon block filters that are better than none. If you can manage to purchase a higher-quality reverse osmosis filtration machine, you will notice the difference rather quickly. What you pay for in quality could save you money in future health costs.

There is an **excellent website to help you determine which filters** may be needed based on your locale (ZIP code) and what is in the waters where you reside. Once you learn more about your local tap water, you can make filtration decisions more clearly. **Go to:** www.ewg.org/tap-water/ whats-in-yourwater.

The Air, the Air—Is Everywhere

You may find this an odd addition to our lifestyle topic, but the air all around us merits greater consideration. Air fills our lungs and enables us to breathe. Air inspires us. It comes in, goes through the blood to every cell, and ultimately leaves, dragging noxious chemicals out with our breath.

Breathing is our way of maintaining our sense of vitality. As a child with asthma, Karilee recalls barely having the energy to move during those times. Ask anyone having trouble breathing how his energy is doing. We all require fresh, vital oxygen to feel our best.

Air, which is mostly nitrogen, was originally made from volcanoes, as burning rocks offered up gases into a new atmosphere. It is something we recycle with our universe surrounding us, as that which has been contained inside the Earth eventually makes its way out.

Those fortunate enough to have spent time near volcanoes, blow holes, or hot mineral springs that bubble from the depths of this Earth can more easily understand our appreciation for such primordial energy.

Mother Nature is a mighty force to reckon with.

Whether we choose to view this from a scientific or spiritual perspective, either way will demonstrate that there is some Force within and around this Earth that is mightier than us humans. As far as we know, always has been and always will be.

Clean air is an essential ingredient for our health and well-being. We simply must become involved in protecting our air, so that we can nourish and replenish our cells. Home air filters are a good place to start. Look for the HEPA technology. Be sure building air systems are regularly cleaned. Next consider putting some attention to improving the air quality at your workplace. Considering air and basic human needs, we're all in this together.

Stress Reduction

No discussion on health and vitality can be comprehensive without discussing stress. Not all of us have stress; only those who are still living. Yet some have more than their share, and others seem to skirt it somehow.

Learning to recognize your own early warning signals is one of the best ways we know to empower yourself. Before we have breakdowns, and meltdowns, we have *downs*. We may experience times of soul loss, when we need soul retrieval.

Take that necessary quiet time every day to hear the beating of your own beautiful heart, your own inner healer, yearning to help this world. Let her come out strong, helping to guide your life.

Listen to the wisdom of your heart before you make big leaps (to avoid finding nothing beneath you). Yes, we all make mistakes. Get over it. Move on. Bless it. Shower the entire experience, and all people involved, with love. Let it go.

Move on to where your own grass grows greener, where Nature calls to you, where you find your place of peace, and power. Do not let the cares of this world crush your soul.

Find your place of peace. Sit carefully, with intention, as you put up your signs, whether physical or just in your mind. "Gone Fishing." "Out to Lunch." "Back Later." Listen to the call of your spirit thirsting for nourishment; heed the calls within.

The Mind-Restoring Bath

- First, make a date with yourself.

Go to your favorite local health food store. Browse; ask for help in learning about essential oils, herbs, and bath products.

Find some natural bath products that are not tainted with heavy chemicals. If you can't pronounce the ingredients, don't buy the product. Smell them, touch them, ask your body which it likes best.

Treat yourself, even if you have to wait for payday or your birthday. Gather your favorite items: oils, bubble bath, powders.

- Now, take a date with yourself:

Turn off phones. Once in the bathroom, lock the door. Put a "Gone Fishin'" sign on your mind.

Sit. Relax. Breathe.

Fill the tub to your desired temperature and level. As it fills, ask your inner self for guidance. Add aromatherapies that suit your immediate needs. You can buy several, rotating them around, allowing your sniffer to make the decisions for now.

Add your favorite natural scents, burn some incense if you like, perhaps even an aroma candle to flicker as you relax.

Call in your Guides. Then create a circle around you to inspire you. It can be Angels you have known, people who have helped to guide your life with their modeling, Jesus, or Mary, or anyone from whom you would like guidance. Put on your favorite soft, relaxing music.

Dim the lights.

Breathe deeply and fully. Listen. Relax. Restore.

- Be with yourself, at last.

This is some of our most important work, and the one we often seem to resist the most!

Spend a few minutes in quiet contemplation.

Ask your Guides to tell you how to move forward in your life. Bless and thank them.

Before ending, set your intention, using affirmations. Remember the power of the carefully spoken word:

"I sleep like a baby and awaken feeling relaxed, restored, and revived."

"I now release anything that no longer serves my highest good. It melts into the water, flowing out and down the drain."

"Peace lives within me, around me, and remains available to me always. I calm my spirit and fill it with Peace."

Then, if you are working toward resolution of some specific large goal, state your intentions for healing.

"Soon this experience will all be behind me."

"Every day, in every way, I'm doing better and better." (Great for recovery)

"When the lesson is received, the messenger can leave."

(Karilee thinks she made this last one up, but can't be sure; she uses it regularly for many life lessons—from financial concerns to relief of bodily symptoms.)

Make each bath special and unique—choose differently each time, honoring the call of your spirit at that moment.

Do this as often as needed to restore your mental wealth.

You'll be glad you did.

Other Stress Busters

Avoid manipulation. Do not, by any means, allow yourself to be manipulated. Choose not to listen to noisemakers, people saying negative things that make you feel worse, even when they are news reporters. If they blabber incessantly, yet say little of value, you need to tune them out. Otherwise, they will drive you to drink.

Learn to set boundaries that objectionable people cannot bridge. Bless them; urge them toward their own healing guides or elsewhere, wherever they do not have power to keep influencing you and others negatively.

When others call you names or put you down, realize it is their own selves they are seeing in your reflection. Because they have refused to accept the gifts offered by self-reflective practices, their toxins spew outward, contaminating those within reach. Without your agreement, they cannot impact you. Know in your heart your own true value and worth.

When they call you "selfish," as generally they will, **they are attempting to make you feel guilty for caring for yourself**.

Do not buy into this manipulation, no matter the source. You can now know, in your heart of hearts, that **what they think or say about you is none of your business**.

> Doing what we need to do for our health and well-being is *not selfish*, nor crazy. It is actually the only sane way to go.

"Stress as a Way of Life" Is Killing Us

We all know it's bad for us. It will kill us if we let it. But do we really know what it *is*?

> Stress is not simply what happens to us. Stress is more about *how we respond* to what happens to us.

Stress reduction is a necessary activity for most of us today, living in our fast-paced world. Time seems to be shrinking while demands grow. Many people today are quickly encouraged to resort to pharmaceutical solutions, without exploring other options. The problems with this approach are many.

Regulatory agencies are unable to stay on top of their oversight, leaving consumers increasingly vulnerable. Absolute reliance on medications outside of ourselves can disempower us, contributing to a sense that we need drugs to live our lives.

Empowered health consumers are discovering a tremendous skill that has been hidden inside of them; a powerful ability to cope and transcend can be reached with adequate support. As we discover this inside us, we are unlikely to resort to medications so frivolously.

Every day there are newly emerging tools coming to the forefront, helping us each to access our own inner healer. Listening to our body and its wisdom is the first, best step to embarking upon our healing journey. Garnering adequate support is the step that ensures we will make it not only today, but also for the long run.

Reduce Your Sources of Stress

- Curtail visits with manipulative people, even if family.
- Take regular time off to rejuvenate.
- Learn to live on less income, and reduce work pressures.
- Opt out of scary movies that tax the adrenal system.
- Consume less caffeine, alcohol, tobacco, and sugar.
- Watch less televised news; it is immune suppressive.
- Reduce your deadline pressures when possible.
- Leave earlier for appointments for less time pressure.
- Say "no" more frequently, rather than overcommit.

Reduce Your Effects from Stress

- Add some slow **stretching**, like yoga, daily.
- Use aerobic **exercise** to burn off excess adrenaline.

- **Self-hypnosis**, affirmations, emotional release, massage, and breathing can help redirect you on a less-stressed path.
- Consider group or individual **counseling** at key times.
- Select only experienced, nonjudgmental therapists.
- Use autogenic training, **part-by-part muscle relaxation**, and eye movement desensitization (EMDR) to destress.
- Chiropractic or osteopathic manipulations can also help.
- **Herbal products** can aid relaxation and stress reduction: valerian, hops, skullcap, lady's slipper, passionflower, orange peel—all are used to calm muscles and mind.
- Tai chi, yoga, qigong, and other **martial arts** have been shown to be very useful for decreasing stress levels.
- There are also ways to let go of the emotional charge of difficult situations, including **writing** it out in journals, and performing **rituals** to release and recharge.
- Using imagery techniques, such as sitting and watching your thoughts pass like daydreams, can be very useful, as well as envisioning positive things happening in your immediate and future times. Keep moving ahead, and expect success.

Mind Power—Restoring the Flow of Hormones

Stress reduction includes a variety of activities such as meditation, self-hypnosis, autogenic training, and many newer forms of these time-honored techniques, which are useful in boosting parasympathetic nervous system tone, lessening the adrenaline-like sympathetic nervous system.

The purpose of stress reduction is to improve and balance the immune function, nervous system, and metabolism, allowing them a chance to cool down in order to perform more effectively.

Decades of experience have convinced us of the untapped power of our minds for creating greater well-being. We feel even more strongly about this now than when Dr. Rich Shames coauthored *Healing with Mind Power* back in the seventies. The integrative health movement relies heavily on the understanding that mind and body are not at all separate. They are simply different aspects of our totality. (Shames)

Philosophers and researchers such as Larry Dossey, MD, have studied *consciousness* for years, helping us to better grasp the concept that mind is a universal experience, as opposed to an interesting attribute of individual collections of brain tissue. It exists, according to quantum theory, as a point of connection for all forms of life.

To have a healthy mind, you need to preserve a healthy body to the best of your abilities. To have a healthy body, you need to maintain a healthy mind. Our integrative explorations have led us to the concept "body-mind." We do not have a body, nor a mind—we have a body-mind.

Hormones are continually flowing back and forth between our various organs and systems. The complexity of our hormonal interaction is truly mind-boggling, yet one thing seems simple and clear. We must have enough of these chemicals to get the job done right. With the right hormone levels, especially the energy-regulating *thyroid hormone*, we can restore our bodies, we can restore our minds, and all together we will notice the improvement in our life.

To reduce your stress levels, **get real** about what you can and can't do. People today are being pushed in their work environments, aiming for more production with less worker cost. Our whole lives seem driven increasingly by the demands of business and finance.

Yet we can always reclaim our lives. We can take that step back, evaluate our position, make better decisions, and do our best without feeling bad that we can't do more. It is not your fault when you cannot complete an inhuman amount of work.

Always do your best; no more, no less.

Learning to not take things personally can provide us with a big leap forward. When we realize how much is out of our control, we can laugh more, lighten up the atmosphere, and simply do our best. We cannot do more without causing ourselves harm. When we restore our thyroid hormones to their full power, life can be truly amazing.

Enjoyable Exercise

Activity is essential: we recommend regular repetitive exercise such as walking, swimming, cycling, rowing, treadmill, NordicTrack, etc. If you do 20 minutes or more 4 or 5 days each week, you are on the road to recovery.

**New research also shows that walking 30 minutes daily can signifi-
cantly reduce women's chances of stroke, a most serious condition.**

Jacob Sattelmair, MSc, of the Harvard School of Public Health,
recently published a study that found during 11.9 follow-up years for the
participants of the Women's Health Study, **walking time and pace were
inversely related to stroke risk** among 40,000 healthy US women age 45
and older. Women who walked 2 hours or more per week, in addition to
having a 30% lower risk for any stroke, were also 57% less likely to have
hemorrhagic stroke.

Getting Started

* When getting started, **stretch well** before and after walking.
* **Stay within your breath** and level of endurance.
* Work up to higher levels gradually, carefully.
* **Listen to your body**; if something has pain, stop.
* **Breathe and rest.** Massage that area gently when possible.
* Begin again slowly, **breathing and releasing** as you walk.

**Some of the best exercise is slow stretching, such as yoga, a very
healing form of movement used for thousands of years.**

Recent years have witnessed an explosion of exercise programs, as
boomers are reaching old age, reluctant to admit it, and seeking ways to
keep our bodies moving and oiled. By now, most of us recognize the need
for movement as a basic human need. Those who are aging seek forms of
exercise that will allow us to live well and prosper.

If you like swimming, keep in mind that many pools have such high
levels of chlorine that it can interfere with thyroid function. So swim moderately, perhaps alternating with other gentle forms of exercise (walking,
cycling, martial arts, dance, and gentle movement).

The Body's Language:
Dance As If No One Is Watching

Many of us love to dance; we hit that floor like some pouncing animal. For
those who relate to this feeling, it may be a lasting remnant of our animal

origins, or not. It may just be that, deep inside, most of us love to dance. Early cultures used dance to release demons, for centuries.

Dance and other movement forms have been used since the earliest shamanic healers, for release and restoration. Before the spoken word, people communicated through movement, using their bodies to tell their stories. Now, lacking movement, our bodies still tell stories on us—not to harm us, rather to support our health. First, we must learn their language.

We can look at certain bodies and know where they are storing energy. We can learn to help each other do what is possible, listening carefully.

When we are energetically compromised, we may not have fortitude to accomplish our dreams. Exercise can help with this, as long as we allow our body-mind to provide us with feedback that we are listening to carefully. Learning to listen to our bodies is one of the critical life skills.

Exercise regularly, within your abilities. Do not further tax your systems with excess "pushing" in your life; instead practice moving within the flow of your life. Learn to stop way before overexertion, which depletes chemicals you need for both the short and the long term.

Listening to your body needs can help you to maintain your health. Learn to listen, to make needed changes. Hearing the call of your body and learning to honor it is the first and most valuable step you can take.

Special Challenges of Thyroid-Types

Many of our patients are highly productive, driven people. Whether they work in academia or on Wall Street, they often exist continually within a cloud of chaos that has become normal to them.

The reality seems to be that today many have become **so addicted to their own adrenaline** that they cannot shut it off, even if their lives depend on doing that. Often, by the time they get to us, their lives do actually depend on their ability to turn off the juice and give it a rest.

This is simply common sense: if you drove your car all day and all night, eventually you would run out of gas. If you drove your body all day and much of the night, it too would eventually slow down.

The Good Book tells us that even the Creator took a day of rest. What hubris we have at times to believe we can keep going endlessly, without doing the same.

When our children were young, we held weekly days of rest, filled with contemplation, writing, laughter, disagreement, and whatever other aspects of our lives needed a voice. These Sabbaths were the one day of the week that everyone stayed in pajamas, and no one went anywhere. Generally they were restful and peaceful times.

We consider to this day that we have provided our offspring with one of the most effective tools available, for free. Learning to rest, relax, regroup, revise, restore, renew, and recharge is part of the holy tradition of many religions. Sabbath is our day of rest.

Honoring this simple tradition was one of the best things we ever did for our growing family. We gave them a sense of creating a balanced life, and how that could feel. Two of our kids loved it; one was adamant as she matured that she wanted to use any time off, not for hanging out at home, but instead for play or work out in the world. We couldn't stop her starting at age 15. Somehow we sense she appreciates our approach more today as she ages.

Listen to Mother Nature Before She Has to Yell

Those who suffer with thyroid imbalance are the canaries in the mines, sensitive ones whose bodies tell us loudly that something within us cannot be sustained. Listening to these voices can help us to recognize even the subtlest forms of danger as they begin to invade our environment. Caring for our own needs is a most basic human activity.

We make choices in life. We can go kicking and screaming, or we can go along enjoying the ride. Some of us do both.

Not everyone wants to keep learning, but those who wish to grow must learn.

We can readily learn from the lessons life provides to us, or we can learn at a very slow pace. It is always our choice.

Just as we can listen to our instincts, we can learn to listen to our bodies. Listen to your body when it calls out to you. Pay attention to the quietest of voices, so your pain does not have to magnify to get your attention.

Prevention gets the best results, by far. Those who live according to Nature's laws live a healthy and balanced life. Listening to the wisdom of our Earth can often stall that time when we shall become her dust.

Bloom where you are planted. Keep your eyes and ears, and especially your heart, open. Live in Love, not fear. Count your blessings. Know your enemies. Do not give in to fear.

We have learned all this, right? But now comes the hard part: remembering, and adhering to these healthful prescriptions, or else.

Lastly, speak your Truth when needed, even if it hurts. In the end, at least you can live with yourself and sleep better at night. That is worth a whole lot. In fact, it could be exactly the medicine called for. And you haven't spent a dime.

Rejuvenating Bodywork

We are amazed when we meet people who do not get any bodywork. To us, it is an essential aspect of our lives. We believe it accounts for a great deal of the good health we both currently enjoy.

Massage—Why We Knead It

Kneading muscles in massage **increases blood and lymph flow**, providing excellent relaxation for healing. Massage helps us to relax, to breathe fully and deeply, to energize and reconnect—body, mind, spirit.

There are many types of bodywork, from gentle Swedish to deeper Rolfing, and everything in between. Most types help us to move more easily back to center, reclaiming a state of comfort and ease, while still living in our temple, the body.

Types of Bodywork

Some massage forms, like Swedish, are very gentle, soft, and flowing, encouraging the muscles to relax and the blood to flow more. Gentle Swedish massage is the type most often provided at health spas. It can certainly add to your relaxation and better mental health.

Any massage can offer better integration, assimilation, and digestion. Results vary depending on the client's ability to relax and breathe as well as the therapist's ability to work within the client's comfort zone.

Another critical influence can relate to the resonance between client and practitioner. If you are not comfortable with a person, do not put yourself in a vulnerable position with him. If, on the other hand, you respect and appreciate the person massaging you, your healing experience will be better.

Deep tissue work with a well-trained professional therapist can help you and loved ones to move those toxins along, out of the blood and lymph, so they can be eliminated. These practitioners are specially trained to work more deeply to enhance elimination by the body. The deeper work helps to reduce built-up adhesions between muscles, tendons, and fascia, helping the body move more smoothly.

It is crucial to drink lots of water after receiving massage, and especially after deep tissue massage. Sometimes people can feel a bit of a headache, a result of toxins releasing through your body. Drink water, plenty of it, and rest. The ideal is to set aside time when you can be fully relaxed, comfortable resting your mind, not on duty for anyone.

Each person is very different. Those with thyroid-related mental symptoms—especially anxiety, depression, nervousness, irritability, rage, or even moderate bodily tension as a result of their thyroid challenge— might wish to try some body therapies. See what helps *you*.

We can only imagine the amazing benefits possible for people with mental disorders after receiving regular massage therapy. As long as we keep writing, we are likely to keep encouraging people feeling "stuck" in their lives to get some really good massage, a great way to get "unstuck."

Not only does it help with our bodies' toxic burdens, but it also can uplift us to that place wherein joy is not only possible, but normal.

A good, seasoned body-worker will know her limits and will elicit feedback when working with painful areas. Always inform your therapist of what your body does and does not handle, or enjoy. Once again, as with many aspects of health, **you are your body's best protector**. Be sure the bodywork is working for you.

It is imperative, if you are the person receiving massage, to do what you can to ensure a healing outcome. Pay attention to your instincts, warn the therapist ahead of time about areas of injury requiring special attention, and be sure to breathe deeply and fully (both the giver and the receiver as well) to help revitalize your body and release toxins more readily.

After experimentation, you will have a better understanding of your body, and what does and does not work for you. We encourage you to consider it your next step to begin to explore what types of bodywork are available in your area.

Be sure to **get specific recommendations** prior to beginning work with a therapist. Do not hesitate to question that person carefully, in a kind way of course, so that you can be sure you have all your concerns addressed. And if, at any time, something is not working for you, make sure you get it to stop. It's your body and your life.

Spiritual Awareness

We were taught in a spiritualist church years ago that there were truly only two basic emotions: Love and Fear. They are said to be different faces of the same person; each of us is continually making choices about which of these faces we will show in the many aspects of our lives.

Clearly, from most religious teachings, we are asked to respond with love first. At times, that can be extremely difficult, but we must persevere.

Our culture today is overladen with so much fear that people are finding less quality and more burnout; adrenals burned younger and younger.

> **Fear, we might recall, is a built-in mechanism that allows us to save our own lives when in danger.**

If we live every minute of every day in fear, where will the creativity be expressed? How can we achieve our life dreams when we live in fear, not knowing where our next meal will come from, or whether we can pay for medical care we may need? We must have faith in order to flip from fear over to love.

A Major Antidote to Feeling "Disconnected"

Spiritual fulfillment in large part determines our eventual overall health. In addition to our basic religious beliefs, there are a number of philosophies and traditions, some arising from the East, that integrative practitioners recommend for enhancing well-being and enjoyment of life.

One of the gifts we can enjoy and give is the pursuit of greater

spiritual connection, no matter what route we take. Our soul longs for this greater joy and deeper understanding. We encourage your active and ongoing participation in whatever feeds your soul.

You may have your own religious practices that help you to trust more in life and to have faith. If these are working well for you, we hope you feel truly blessed. Not everyone, however, settles comfortably into an organized religion they can believe in wholeheartedly.

Some people feel a need to develop more of an individual spirituality, to feel their own personal connection with their own "Higher Power." Learning to make this connection can often mean the difference between faith and fear—or even life and death.

Connecting to Our Spirit

Spirituality keeps us connected, each within our self, one to another, and to our world. Many of us feel some force that guides our lives, even if we are not sure how to describe it. Not everyone needs it defined.

Modern feminist author bell hooks suggests dangers arise if we turn from love. **Love** is this mystical aspect that is very hard to live without in our present world. Spiritual practices, whether of an organized religion, mindfulness meditation, or spirit guide visualization, help us to grow and connect to our higher power.

There is no disease so prominent today in our culture as that of loneliness and alienation. Many people are living quiet lives of desperation, often isolated from their loved ones and separated from their deepest strength. They have in some respects lost their way.

Spirituality is the way home, to our hearts, to our health, to our Love. It is an opening of the heart that allows Grace to enter, and Fear to leave.

As holistic practitioners, we do not only consider that we are body-mind; what we see is that we are a unity of body-mind-spirit.

Healing can occur through the spirit, mind, or body. For these reasons, we seek not only to use vitamins and hormones but also to inspire you to release, to laugh, to play, to love, to cry, to gather, to pray.

Especially as we gather, Miracles occur, and Love heals us further.

(For those seeking a more philosophical view, see Karilee's Afterword.)

Complementary Healing for Your Best Results

By Georjana Shames, LAc

In Chapters 4 through 8, you read about *specific* Chinese Medicine guidance for the different Five Elements types of people. Now please enjoy these lifestyle suggestions in the form of *general* tips for regulating your thyroid to improve overall mental health. Since proper sleep, strong digestion, good diet, and life balance all factor heavily in mental health, you will find many of those aspects addressed below.

REST, SLEEP, AND INSOMNIA

Two hours before bedtime, dim all the lights in your house and turn off phones and computers. Enjoy a hot bath, read, and relax.

Remember that compared to the long arc of human history, it has only been in the past century or so that electricity has become widely available. For perhaps millions of years prior to that, humans were generally retiring soon after sunset. There was little else to keep us awake and distracted.

- Just 15 minutes of **sunshine** per day raises your vitamin D levels, boosting your mood and immune function.

- Try taking more **rest and relaxation** (even if you have to force yourself). Rejuvenation for body and mind is worth its weight in gold! You will be productive more of the time if you rest some of the time.

FOOD

- Boost your heart health by **eating plenty of vegetables**, legumes, and whole grains. Enjoy plenty of brown rice, brightly colored vegetables (bell peppers and beets), greens, yams, lean meats, and veggie sprouts.

- **Lose weight** by eliminating dairy, white flour, and excess sugars from your diet. Start with dairy because in Chinese Medicine dairy creates what we call "Dampness," which causes excess weight. I ask my patients, "When was the last time you went to a Chinese restaurant and saw cheese or butter or cream on the menu?" It is unheard of.

- In the Chinese way, **avoiding dairy** is ideal. However, goat dairy creates less Dampness than cow dairy. If you must have some, grate small amounts of goat cheese over your meals. Eat your cereal with almond milk, pour rice milk in your tea, and learn to minimize cow dairy products.

- If you suffer from abdominal distension and pain, eat five organic strawberries prior to each meal.
- In Chinese Medicine what we call a Blood deficiency can certainly lead to depression. **Boosting your red blood cells** can help build the Blood. Especially if you are anemic, add beets, black beans, black sesame seeds, organic meat, and dark leafy veggies to your diet.
- Many thyroid patients suffer from tinnitus (ringing in the ears). Drinking a tea made of **chrysanthemum flowers** daily can help reduce annoying sound.
- Many of those with autoimmune thyroiditis suffer from seasonal allergies as well. For allergies—especially with mild coughing—twice daily take a small spoonful of **local honey** and place at the back of the throat to dissolve. Local honeybees ingest and process the pollens that exist in your area; if you consume the resulting honey, it can help eliminate allergies. Also, honey coats the throat to reduce friction and irritation.

EXERCISE
Remember to do something **fun** for your **exercise** so that you will absolutely stick to it, whether that is dance, biking, hiking, yoga, or running down the street after your untrained dog, pulling the leash.

STAY STRONG
- To **avoid colds**: wear a scarf to protect the occipital area at the back of the neck (called "The Wind Gate" in Chinese Medicine).
- Balancing your thyroid will **boost your immune function**, leaving you less susceptible to every cold and flu that goes around. If you do get a cold or flu that turns into bronchitis, steam several cored Asian pears for 30 minutes; eat the whole fruit with a spoonful of local honey drizzled on it.

TAME THOSE ADDICTIONS
- **Quitting smoking** is one of the best things you can do for your health. To quit and stay off cigarettes forever, make sure you cultivate good habits to replace the smoking habit (like exercise, writing or sketching, meditation, Acupuncture for addiction).

   You can begin by snipping one end off all your cigarettes, decreasing the length of each by about one-fourth. Immediately, you have cut down on your smoking habit (as long as you do not increase the number of cigarettes you use—no cheating now!). Soon you can snip more off each cigarette, decreasing by one-third, then one-half, and so on.

ENJOY!

When all is said and done, please know that we wish you success and blessings on your healing journey. May you touch many lives with your inspiration, and may the infinite life force be with you always.

THE BOTTOM LINE

- Your lifestyle choices are central to what happens to your health.
- These are the categories of revitalization we recommend:
  — Sensible nutrition

  — Stress reduction

  — Enjoyable exercise

  — Rejuvenating bodywork

  — Spiritual growth
- **Optimal thyroid status** can help you meet your full potential. Full recovery can be the greatest gift you have ever received.
- Thyroid treatment, natural or by prescription, is much more effective when **combined with targeted lifestyle enhancements**.
- **Eat organic** when possible, which allows for less toxic buildup in your body and on the planet.
- People with less thyroid function often digest much too slowly, resulting in lower health. **Keep your bowels flowing**; eat fiber.
- Thyroid types need a food **intake low in calories**, meats, and dairy and **high in vegetables, fruits, seeds, nuts, and sprouts**.
- In and around the house, **be wary of using any synthetic chemicals**, as they are frequently hormone disrupters.
- Learn to **use food, clean water, and other lifestyle modifications as your best defense** against illness.
- **Find your place of peace, often.** Calm your spirit so you can make your best decisions. Listen carefully. Be courageous.
- **Stress** is not so much what happens to us; it is more about *how we respond* to what happens. **Learn to live with less stress.**

- **Prevention** gets best results, and avoids a whole lot of problems. Relieving internal stress is a great way to keep hormones flowing.

- **Massage** can offer better integration, assimilation, and digestion. Try various types of bodywork, and keep using those that seem most appropriate for your particular health issues.

- No disease is so prominent in our culture as that of loneliness, and alienation. **Connecting is the antidote.** Explore your own personal spiritual path with devotion and commitment.

- **Enjoy each day of your life as the gift it is.** Revel, laugh, and play often. Make more time for those you love, including yourself. And your pet. Your family and your hobbies. Life can be a gas! Enjoy.

RECOMMENDED ACTION PLAN

- Know that your lifestyle choices have a huge impact on your long-term approach to successful thyroid balance.

- Strive to upgrade your nutrition, stress reduction, and exercise programs.

- To improve your nutrition program:

  — Avoid fatty or fried foods, too much salt or spice; **eat lightly and gently**.

  — Avoid chlorine and fluoride.

  — **Eat less meat, especially grilled meats**, and seek more organic, nonchemical meats and foods.

  — Chew well.

  — Go easy on the alcohol!

  — Eat less **sugar, chocolate**, and stimulants, including **coffee**.

  — Avoid **synthetic chemicals** in products you use.

- To reduce your sources of stress:

  — Curtail visits with **manipulative people**, even if family.

  — Take regular **time off** to rejuvenate.

  — Learn to **live on less** income to reduce work pressure.

  — **Opt out of scary movies** that tax the adrenal system.

  — Consume **less caffeine,** alcohol, tobacco, and sugar.

  — Watch **less televised news**; too much may be immune suppressive.

  — Reduce your **deadline pressures** when possible.

- — Leave earlier for appointments for **less time pressure**.

- — **Say "no"** more frequently, rather than overcommit.

- To reduce your effects of stress:

  - — Try more daily **stretching**, such as yoga. Breathe fully.

  - — Use aerobic **exercise** to burn off excess adrenaline.

  - — Experiment with **self-hypnosis**, affirmations, emotional release, massage, and breathing exercises to help foster a less-stressed path.

  - — Consider group or individual **counseling** at key times.

  - — Select only experienced, **nonjudgmental therapists**.

  - — Use autogenic training, **part-by-part muscle relaxation**, and eye movement desensitization (EMDR) to de-stress.

  - — **Chiropractic** or osteopathic manipulations can also help.

  - — **Herbal products** aid relaxation: valerian, hops, skullcap, lady's slipper, passionflower, and orange peel—all calm muscles and mind.

  - — Tai chi, yoga, qigong, and other **martial arts** have been shown to be very useful for decreasing stress levels.

  - — There are also ways to let go of the emotional charge of difficult situations, including **journaling** or rituals for release and recharge.

  - — Get real about what you can and can't do. Get **therapy** as needed.

  - — Set boundaries; be assertive and clear.

- To upgrade your exercise program:

  - — **Stretch well** before and after exercise. Stay within your breath and level of endurance. Work up to higher levels gradually, carefully.

  - — Listen to your body. **Exercise regularly** within your own abilities.

The Program in a Nutshell

Step One: Consider a Thyroid *Cause*

Chapter 1: Thyroid conditions are **extremely common and often misdiagnosed**, causing a wide variety of symptoms.

Begin to see **beyond** the **artificial distinction of mind and body** as separate aspects. You are one whole connected person. Everything affects all else.

Chapter 2: Realize that **thyroid issues can be the root cause** of *any* long-standing psychological issues.

Know that **optimal treatment of thyroid imbalance** can provide additional **relief** from depression, anxiety, loss of memory and focus, sleep problems, and harmful habits.

Chapter 3: Know that you could still be thyroid imbalanced, even with "normal" results on regular blood tests.

Choose the new and **more accurate panel of finger-stick blood tests**, available at www.CanaryClub.org under "Thyroid Tests."

Be sure to **take the questionnaire**. Be very *suspicious* for thyroid diagnosis if you have significant symptoms, family history, related conditions, or physical signs.

Now begin your ongoing "Jump Start" (with Metagenics items):

- Multivitamins (Multigenics—four daily in AM)
- Antioxidants (Oxygenics—one daily in AM)
- Omega oils (Omega-EFA—one daily in AM)
- Amino acids (BioPure Protein—one scoop daily)

Step Two: Understand Your Best *Treatment*

Each chapter in this step provides specific suggestions for one particular kind of mental symptoms. Choose the one chapter that represents your most urgent area of concern. That chapter's suggested items can now be *added* to your morning daily jump start.

Regarding the suggestions below, begin each new item *one at a time for 5 days*, to be sure you tolerate it well. After 5 days, you can add the next item from that chapter. *If anything does not feel right, stop taking it* and move on to other suggestions from that same chapter. (Additional items for your long-term thyroid balancing will be available later, in Step Three.)

Chapter 4: For over-the-counter treatment of thyroid-related depression, start with a mixed thyroid booster containing **standardized rosemary extract** (like two pills daily of Thyrosol from Metagenics).

After 5 days, add a high-quality **vitamin D** (such as two pills daily of Iso D₃ from Metagenics).

If this is not adequately helpful after a month, *add* a stepwise increasing trial of **prescription desiccated thyroid**, such as Armour or Nature-Throid, from a qualified practitioner.

Chapter 5: For over-the-counter treatment of the Edgy mind-type, start with a high-quality **balanced thyroid glandular** (such as two pills daily of T-150 from Xymogen).

After 10 days, add **evidence-based thyroid-boosting nutrients** (like three pills daily of MedCaps T3 by Xymogen).

If this is not adequately helpful after 1 month, *add* a stepwise increasing trial of **prescription levothyroxine** (T4 thyroid hormone), from a qualified practitioner.

Companies like Lannett, Sandoz, and Mylan make high-quality generic levothyroxine that is easily as good as the more expensive brand names.

Chapter 6: For over-the-counter treatment of thyroid-related memory and focus issues, start first with bioactive amounts of **guggulsterone** (such as two pills daily of Lipotain by Metagenics).

After 5 days, you may enhance the effectiveness of guggul's thyroid boosting with an extra-strong, well-tolerated **antioxidant** (like one pill daily of Oraxinol by Xymogen).

If this is not adequately helpful after a month, *add* a stepwise increasing trial of straight prescription liothyronine (**T3 thyroid hormone**). This can be brand name Cytomel, generic T3, or timed-release T3 from a compounding pharmacy.

Chapter 7: For over-the-counter treatment of thyroid-related sleep problems, start with five pellets dissolved under the tongue three times daily of the homeopathic remedy **Coffea Cruda** (for high thyroid) or **Thyroidinum** (for low thyroid). You can find these at a good vitamin store. Ask for the 6 or 12 potency, and use for *only 2 weeks,* then stop.

If you do not feel adequately improved after a month, then *add* a stepwise increasing trial of **prescription T3/T4 combo** from a qualified practitioner. This is best accomplished with *two* separate bottles of medicine, one of T4 (levothyroxine), the other of T3 (liothyronine).

Chapter 8: For over-the-counter help with thyroid-related harmful habits, start with the strong herbal medicine *Withania somnifora*, commonly called **ashwaganda**. (Try two pills twice daily of Mentalin by Metagenics.)

After 5 days, boost its effectiveness with an **amino acid and thyroid support** formula (such as three tablets daily of Energenics by Metagenics).

If this is not fully successful, combine it with a trial of **prescription compounded levothyroxine** (T4 thyroid hormone) from a qualified practitioner, sending your prescription to a compounding pharmacy (www.pccarx.com).

Step Three: Maintain a Lasting *Cure*

Chapter 9: Keep an **open mind**. Any thyroid-balancing program can be further improved with additional supportive vitamins and minerals, herbal medicines, appropriate enzymes, attention to the underlying autoimmune issue, and focus on related medical/hormonal concerns. Extra iodine, for example, is sometimes useful, but sometimes best avoided.

Make your **long-term maintenance** *personal* and *individualized* from the many options offered. Choose items that feel consistent with your wallet, beliefs, and interests.

Chapter 10: Know that your *lifestyle choices* have a huge impact on your long-term approach to successful thyroid balance. Strive to upgrade your **nutrition, stress reduction**, and **exercise** programs.

Be sure to include some relaxing **bodywork**, but especially pay closer attention to the messages of your body, and to your **spiritual growth**. This can be extremely life enhancing.

Afterword

Beyond These Three Steps: "Meeting at the Mountaintop"

By Karilee Shames, PhD, RN

In this final section, I seek to step out of the medical model a bit further.

As a holistic nurse, I enjoy more freedom in helping clients learn to listen to messages sent by their bodies.

With due respect to the many incredible physicians practicing with skill and devotion, it long ago became clear to me that if nursing is to take its proper place in the medical hierarchy, nursing must provide gifts to our patients that doctors often do not. The difference is huge and worthy of your attention.

Today's nurses are busting out of traditional roles, working alongside doctors, nurse practitioners, physician assistants, nutritionists, body-workers, energy healers, shamanistic healers, and more. Many have prepared for years to assist you in becoming well and living fully.

Holistic nursing teaches us to develop a sense of appreciation for the interconnectedness of the diverse aspects of our being. We are physical beings, capable of expanding and growing through spiritual awakenings.

We have desires, dreams, and aspirations. When we follow them, we each discover our Higher Power. Our visions become our lives when we learn to work within the laws of nature (I call them the Laws of Mother Nature).

When we are not paying close attention or when we refuse to learn, we are slowed in our progress by forces that often arise outside of us—including beliefs, arbitrary rules, and hungry humans. Any of these can detract us from our fondest dreams. Integrative nurses can help to guide you in your life.

Nurses can be instrumental in helping you to reclaim your soul before you lose your will. We can advise you so that you can be aware of potential dangers. Ultimately, you must care for yourself. No one can heal you, except you.

Becoming Your Own Best Healer

One of my favorite exercises with clients is to have them simply sit and listen to their body as it speaks to them. In this form of visualization, I walk them through as they touch parts of their own bodies, breathing fully and deeply together, awakening body parts and the emotions they may hold within.

Over decades, having studied ancient and modern modalities, I found that **people often need support and guidance to become their own best healers**. One of the ways you can do this is to begin eating cleaner foods, as well as doing your best to clean your life in as many arenas as possible. One book that I deeply appreciate is called *Cellular Cleansing Made Easy,* by Scott Ohlgren. This program walks you through steps to reduce your symptoms, replenish needed items, and regenerate your cells. It is a perfect next step to follow our book and program.

And our most valuable recommendation, in addition to cleansing and eating well, would be to take at least 1 day off each week. If the Lord needs a day of rest, what could possibly excuse our forgetting to rest? This is a critical aspect of healing.

Embrace the Big Positives and Avoid the Great Detractors

Beliefs can be thoughts we have adopted from an early age. They may have been helpful at one time, or never truly helpful. They guide us in our lives toward the Light when helpful, and away from the Light when not.

Rules are necessary for people to live with order in a society. Our laws and rules are only as good as the minds of the people we have empowered to create and enforce them. We must choose our leaders very wisely, trusting our own instincts above the advice of others.

Hungry humans are those who suck up our energy and our joy, trying to make us feel unhappy because they resent our happiness. This is frequently not a pretty picture; those of us who seek the mountaintop must learn to avoid detractors along the journey. Most of us are content to live within the laws of nature, and of our society. There have always been some, however, who choose to believe they are above these laws, who allow their greed to direct their behaviors.

These hungry humans recall *The Hungry Thing*, a children's book about a monster that comes to town and starts eating up everything in sight. This is not a bad monster, just a voracious one. But hungry humans can wreak terrible havoc on our lives.

Many people have been injured in their lives, often in ways that are very difficult to correct. Without proper skills and support, these people have been doomed to lives of despair. These wounded people may also act out in their rage, causing those around them to suffer due to their inner pain, projected outward.

They often do not mean to hurt you; they simply are desperate to feel better. Anyone in their path can become a victim, if they are not paying attention.

You may recognize this description; you may have even been a hungry human at one time. The good news is that you can reshape the way you think and redesign your life. But you will need help.

The hungry wolf ate Little Red Riding Hood. Did we really grasp that story as children? As we mature, we do seem to encounter hungry wolves, often in sheep's clothing. It is up to us to tell the difference.

Use Your Gifts to Guide Your Life

Most of us humans come fully equipped. As long as we maintain our bodies and do not unduly stress them, we pretty much have everything we need to be successful. One of the greatest internal gifts is our intuition.

Intuition is a high-level activation of our five senses. If we are really listening, and if we allow our senses to feed us information (truly tasting, smelling, seeing, and hearing, as well as touching), something special happens. When we are open to feedback from all our senses, a sixth sense synergistically kicks in. This sixth sense is often referred to as intuition.

One of the bigger challenges we thyroid types face is that our symptoms can look like many other syndromes. Fatigue; depression; overweight; poor digestion; sluggish brain; headaches; pain syndromes; muscle aches; dry hair, skin, and nails . . . the list goes on and on. Slowed or disrupted thyroid metabolism can look a lot like other conditions. It can also mirror the symptoms of body toxicity.

Listening to our intuition and **learning to come back to the wisdom of our bodies is one of the most magnificent gifts we can receive.**

Our lives are a gift from the Universe; enjoying them is our way of giving back to Her.

Life can be very demanding at times, challenging in ways that can break our spirits. But when we learn to ignite our own self-healing abilities, we can fix almost anything. You are not broken, simply malfunctioning. With the proper tools, you can fix your life.

Tools for Your Journey

We have already discussed many ways for you to reclaim your thyroid health and mental well-being. Here, I wish to share some subtle gifts you can learn to give yourself, approaches to your life that will make it even more full of health, joy, and ease.

1. Discernment: Own Your Power to Make Better Decisions.

To discern means to be able to tell the difference between things. Some things are healthy for us; others are not. Some people are true friends; others are only pretending to be for their own purposes.

To maintain ongoing health, you need to be able to tell the difference. If you think chocolate—or beer—loves you, are you willing to face a possible addiction in order to get to the truth? If not, you are dealing with an addiction that has a powerful grasp on your life. If so, stop using the substance for 4 days or more and see how you feel.

Most people feel better when they stop taking something that has negative effects. First you may go through a few days of feeling worse; that is natural and to be expected as your body attempts to clean it out. Then, after 72 hours or more, you should begin to feel great.

The same holds for cutting out people who are not working in your life. You may have tried, for years even, to work with them, but always end up feeling drained. These folks cannot be your true friends; they are fighting their own inner demons. Sometimes the best gift you can provide for them, and for you, is to let go for a while.

Teach your children, well, to listen to their own inner guidance. Ask them to tell you when something does not feel right, and listen carefully to them.

2. Authenticity: Be True, Trustworthy, Genuine, and Original.

When we are authentic, we give of our deepest selves. We offer our love (when it feels right to do so); we withhold our love when it does not feel safe to give it. We speak from a place of truth deep in our hearts, sharing what we believe, even when that may not be a popular view.

When we give of our authentic selves, we are activating our own channels of flow in our lives. We are allowing our hormones to move in the directions they must move, speaking freely, guided by love. Love is the power that heals; it heals every aspect of our lives when we allow it to do so.

Hormones are an intricate aspect of this system, flowing forth in proper amounts at the right times, guided by love. When we are angry, upset, feeling unloved or unlovable, our hormones cannot be in balance.

The more "in balance" we can be in our lives, the more our hormones will flow to where they are needed.

Think of balance as the finish line, and allow yourself to cross that line many times each day.

In fact, every time you envision yourself, see yourself as crossing that finish line.

Allowing yourself to live in that balance more and more of each day will improve the quality of your life enormously. Make the decision to stop giving power to events and people that upset you; instead find your sacred place of authenticity, balance, and love, and hang there.

3. Creativity: Allow Your Life Force to Flow like a Fountain.

To be creative is to make imaginative use of resources available. When we are living in our authentic selves, our creativity flows without our having to put conscious attention to it. Expressing yourself through creativity can yield countless rewards.

4. Integrity and Honesty: Speak Your Truth.

Never doubt that any committed person can make a difference. We have already been shown that we can. Our task is to allow our truth to guide our lives.

You may win more "friends" with conformity, but you are not being your best friend when you do not share what is true for you. Anyone can lie, and many do. You are the only person who can share your truth with this world. If you do not share your heart, who will?

Integrity is the quality of possessing and adhering to high moral principles. While we are all given people who try to influence us to their ways of thinking, what is really true for you is what arises from within, not what you hear from without.

While you may learn many things, to be certain you are being honest, your teachings must be passed through the filter of the heart. If you hear it and it attracts you, if you run it through your heart and it resonates as true for you, then you are living in integrity.

5. Awareness: Listen, Observe, Recall, Transform.

There is a saying: "If you snooze, you lose."

There is another saying: "You can lose, but don't lose the lesson."

From this perspective, our entire life can look so different. We see beyond the obvious and learn to see with new eyes. We trust in the infinite grace of our journey and allow doors to open at last.

The neighbor who has made it impossible for us to live comfortably may have opened doors we would never have seen. The teacher who failed us may have encouraged us to reach out for something better. The lover who left may have allowed us, at long last, to find our truest love.

Being aware means moving through your life with all eyes open wide, all ears listening carefully, and all senses alert and active. We have so many capacities that we may have ignored, with society's encouragement. Now, finally, we can return to the inner strengths, those that spoke to us as children and now want to be revisited.

Your heart knows its truth; can you hear it speaking as it beats? Your eyes within, can you open them? Your ears can hear beyond the noise. Listen carefully.

6. Gratitude: The Final Lift to Heaven's Gate.

Your slow metabolism may have brought you to this place. You have within you the ability to move so far beyond it.

Take precious time, every day, to center, to listen, to love.

Hear the calling of your life, and move back into Balance.

Follow your path, using all the tools you have been given.

Learn from every person you meet, even the hungry humans; bless them, and move forward.

And when we meet, if I have lost my way, your being is all I need.

In your presence, I am reminded of all that I am.

Heaven is within our shared consciousness. We are one.

In gratitude I continue this journey with you, on love's wings.

Appendix

Self-Ordering Your Own Accurate Thyroid Tests

High-quality, low-cost thyroid testing is available for you to self-order through a recently developed health advocacy group called the Canary Club (www.CanaryClub.org).

With your no-cost membership, you receive a special rate on testing panels. You may self-order a home test kit, which will be mailed to you by a top-rated lab. You merely follow the instructions for sample collection, and then send your specimens back to the lab in a prepaid mailer. Results of the testing will be sent to you, along with an interpretation guide.

In our view, **the club's ZRT panel is the easiest, least expensive, and most accurate thyroid testing available to the general public.**

ZRT Lab is a highly-certified hormone-testing laboratory in Beaverton, Oregon. It was established in 1998 and is independently owned and operated by David T. Zava, PhD, a biochemist and breast cancer researcher.

The ZRT thyroid panel that you order contains determinations for Free T4, Free T3, TSH, and thyroid peroxidase (TPO) antibody. This testing is more comprehensive than what the average practitioner will order, and you do not need your doctor's permission to obtain it.

An abnormal result on any of the four tests means you are very likely to have thyroid imbalance.

Further interpretation guidance is available in the "Interpretting Results" section (under After-Testing) of the Canary Club website. Keep in mind:

> **Borderline high or borderline low levels are suspicious for thyroid abnormality.**

Tests should be interpreted *along with your Chapter 3 questionnaire* results.

If you are unsure as to the actual meaning of your test panel, you should discuss your results with a qualified practitioner. If you prefer, you may arrange for a telephone appointment with a Canary Club–recommended licensed medical expert or one of this book's authors.

Our Testing Recommendations

For those who wish **Thyroid-Only** testing, start with ZRT Lab's "Thyroid Panel." This includes:

- TSH
- Free T4
- Free T3
- TPO antibody

For those who wish to have a 12-test panel (**thyroid, adrenal, sex hormones**), order ZRT Lab's "AdvancedPlus Panel." This includes:

- All of the Thyroid-Only tests mentioned above
- Four samples for DHEA and cortisol levels
- Estrogen, progesterone, testosterone, and vitamin D levels

For those who wish to use a doctor-ordered standard blood draw at a local lab, the panel for your practitioner to request should include:

- TSH
- Free T4
- Free T3
- TPO antibody
- Thyroglobulin antibody

Note: Have your doctor order this exact panel at a lab near you by writing it on a lab request slip.

For those who wish to **self-order** our highly recommended thyroid panel, go to www.CanaryClub.org.

Finding and Working with Thyroid-Friendly Practitioners

If you are unable to schedule with us, we urge you to utilize any suggestions in this book in the context of working with a practitioner you trust and enjoy. If you do not have such a health professional, talk to people in your own community to try to locate your best options for doctors and other practitioners. Many people find help in local group meetings, where this information can be shared confidentially.

To be honest, after years in practice, we are well aware that many thousands of you are not being listened to adequately. We hope to help change that.

You deserve to be heard.

Here, we have provided tools for your **Empowerment**.

- We want you to be bold in asking for what you would like to have, including tests, treatments, and respect.
- If you are not getting adequate care, we encourage you to expand your health options.
- If you are feeling discounted by your doctor, or simply cannot get your doctor to order specific tests, it may be time to make necessary changes.
- We encourage you as health consumers to be courageous and bold in your health goals, and to find excellent practitioners to help you meet those goals.
- Nurse practitioners, integrative nurse specialists, physician assistants, osteopathic doctors, naturopathic doctors, chiropractors, acupuncturists, nutritionists, professional body-workers, individual and family therapists, and many others are available to help you reclaim your health, body-mind-spirit.
- You have the right to retain copies of all your evaluations; you have the right to know what is included in your medical chart.
- And, in our view, you have the right to work with any practitioners you choose.

Part of being proactive is to make sure you are working with good practitioners, experienced in this open-minded and interactive manner, and willing to consider your input very carefully.

To that end, we have considered all mind-types in terms of how they may relate to doctors based on their symptoms and related behaviors. This may help you to understand a little more about how to initiate the process of improving your doctor-patient relationship.

What to Show Your Doctor

We have spoken with people from all over the country. They have generally relayed to us that their practitioners, particularly alternative ones, seem to be interested in books, magazine articles, and newsletters, as well as references to scientific literature.

Medical doctors, however, seem to be unmoved by anything except citations and articles from the medical literature. By "medical literature" we mean articles from peer-reviewed journals—the more well known the better.

It is our advice to you, the reader, to bring in and show to your practitioner only those items that will appeal to the practitioner favorably (i.e., only medical journal articles for MDs, and appropriate related material for other health practitioners).

OUR RECOMMENDATIONS FOR ENSURING
THE BEST POSSIBLE RESPONSE

- Do not show your medical doctor our book, or any other books, unless they are **medical textbooks**.
- Never show an MD anything from a newspaper, magazine, or—above all—the Internet (unless you can produce a downloaded copy of an **article or abstract from a medical journal**).
- In general, we suggest searching for something in the chiropractic literature for chiropractors, in acupuncture literature for acupuncturists, and above all, **stick to medical journal references** for medical doctors.

We have provided a sampling of books and websites that can help you get started on your search for the most appropriate materials to show your practitioner. You may need to fish through these, but if you take the time to do this well, it will greatly improve your chances for success in communicating with your practitioner.

Once you have shown your practitioner the journal article (properly highlighted regarding your specific needs), then ask your practitioner if he or she can work creatively with your individual situation to best address these concerns. Ideally you would have options and be able to work with someone who agrees to be supportive.

Is Your Current Doctor Right for *You*?

1. Is your doctor courteous to you, and supportive in general?

2. Does your doctor inspire you to do your best to improve your health?

3. Is your doctor responsive and helpful with your anxieties, willing to answer your questions prior to procedures or prescriptions?

4. Does your doctor present current research and valuable information?

5. Does your doctor do a thorough job of physical, mental, emotional, and possibly even spiritual assessment in addition to relying on blood tests?

6. Is your doctor willing to view you as an individual, perhaps with your own unique ranges of normal for certain tests?

7. Does your doctor generally present concerns about your health in a positive manner (one that avoids blaming you for your health problems and avoids providing the scariest worst-case scenarios immediately)?

8. Does your doctor seem interested and act supportive when you mention vitamins or other natural protocols?

9. Will your doctor review materials you've brought in from your own research, such as a medical journal article or a respected health book?

10. Does your doctor view you as an equal partner in your health care team?

11. Does your doctor answer your questions to your satisfaction, without leaving you feeling dismissed or brushed off?

12. Does your doctor ask about your wishes, preferences, and beliefs prior to coming up with a plan?

13. Will your doctor sign prescription slips to refer you to complementary practitioners of your choice?

14. Are the staff members in your doctor's office respectful and helpful, and is the environment conducive to healing?

15. Has your doctor been forthright and cooperative about your requests for ancillary treatments?

SCORING YOUR QUESTIONNAIRE

If you answered no to three or more of these questions, we recommend that you consider "shopping" for a better match. For some people, including those who are especially sensitive, having even one "no" answer in the list above could be sufficient to warrant a reconsideration of your primary and related practitioners. Do what is right for *your* health.

Finding Your Recommended Vitamins

Out of the hundreds of companies and thousands of products available, we have found the greatest thyroid-rebalancing success with the companies **Metagenics, Inc.**, and **Xymogen**. We can assure you these are some of the highest-grade nutraceutical (pharmaceutical-grade) products available.

Recently we have added two more companies to our list after excellent experiences with their products. These include **Enzymes, Inc.**, and **Naturally Vitamins**. Recommendations for these products are largely provided in Chapter 9.

Below, we tell you more about each company and how best to order their products. (Authors disclose a fiduciary relationship with these companies where there is one.) For more information, please visit www.ThyroidMindPower.com.

Metagenics, Inc.

The company was founded in 1983 with the mission to improve health by helping people achieve their genetic potential through nutrition. Metagenics is located in San Clemente, California, with its world-class functional medicine research center in Gig Harbor, Washington. Through special arrangement, consumers can directly access these products after being educated and advised by us. **You need to tell them you are following Dr. Shames's protocol to order.**

> To purchase Metagenics products:
> Call 1-800-692-9400.
> Be sure to tell them you are following **Dr. Shames's** protocol.

Xymogen

This company has nearly 3 decades of experience in providing exclusive professional formulas to health practitioners. Xymogen is dedicated to the highest quality, with all products tested by third-party lab assay. Now, through special arrangement, consumers can access these products after being educated and advised by us. **You must tell them you are following Dr. Shames's protocol to order.**

> To purchase Xymogen products:
> Call 1-800-647-6100.
> Remember to tell them you are following **Dr. Shames's** protocol.

Enzymes, Inc.

Formulating high-quality products for health professionals, Enzymes, Inc., has come a long way since 1932, when Dr. Edward Howell introduced the first nutritional enzyme support. Now the company has an extensive family of enzyme-based blends, some combined with herbs and other nutrients, to assist discriminating practitioners and their patients with a wide variety of health concerns.

> To purchase Enzymes, Inc., products:
> Call 1-800-637-7893.
> Remember to tell them you are following **Dr. Shames's** protocol.

Naturally Vitamins

With more than 60 years of industry experience, this company is a leader in innovative health care solutions. Its production facility, Marlyn Pharmaceuticals, far exceeds the national GMP (good manufacturing practices) standards, operating under the guidelines of the United States Pharmacopoeia (USP).

> To purchase Naturally Vitamins products:
> Call 1-800-899-4499.
> Remember to tell them you are following **Dr. Shames's** protocol.

EcoNugenics

Within this book, we have also described and suggested products from EcoNugenics.

> To purchase EcoNugenics products:
> Call 1-800-308-5518.
> Tell them that **Dr. Shames** referred you.

Resources

There are many resources available to help you move beyond your thyroid issues.

A good place to start is our own new website, www.ThyroidMindPower .com, where you will find additional diagnostic and treatment information, referrals to other resources, as well as ways to contact our office for tele- phone coaching or in-person appointments.

For those interested in learning more about complementary healing and Chinese Medicine, please take advantage of the information provided by Georjana Shames on her websites: www.ShamesHealth.com and www. ThyroidAcupuncture.com (or contact her directly at 415–388–0456):

- View videos on Acupuncture for hormone balancing and mental/ emotional health.
- Learn more about how this ancient medicine benefits you in the modern world.
- Make appointments for in-person or telephone sessions with Geor- jana Shames, LAc, DiplOM, CMT.

We do encourage you all to join www.CanaryClub.org and send others to be tested and further educated about current thyroid issues. In addition to ordering your testing, the Canary Club posts articles and hosts confer- ence calls to keep you well informed. We do conference calls via Canary Club, too.

One recent development has been www.DearThyroid.org, which lists a variety of resources and options for you to consider. Through this group, you can gather with those similarly affected, sharing in a very creative and healing manner.

We also suggest that you read any or all of Mary Shomon's excellent thyroid books, especially for those who seek greater depths in the science and research.

Each practitioner group (osteopaths, chiropractors, naturopaths, and so forth) will often have its own website, many helping you to access local caregivers in that field.

SUMMARY OF HELPFUL WEBSITES

www.ThyroidMindPower.com (Information and office website for Richard and Karilee Shames)

www.ShamesHealth.com (The website of acupuncturist Georjana Shames)

www.Thyroid-Info.com (Great resource for all things thyroid, from health advocate Mary Shomon)

www.CanaryClub.org (Resource for your best testing options)

www.DearThyroid.org (Provides support and opportunities to write your story)

www.FluorideAlert.org (Everything you never knew about fluoridation—be sure to read why EPA professionals oppose fluoride at www.FluorideAlert.org/hp-epa.htm)

www.HolisticMedicine.org (American Holistic Medical Association)

www.AHNA.org (American Holistic Nurses Association)

www.acatoday.com (American Chiropractic Association)

www.aoa-net.org (American Osteopathic Association)

info@amtamassage.org (American Massage Therapy Association)

www.Naturopathic.org (American Association of Naturopathic Physicians)

www.pccarx.com (Professional Compounding Centers of America)

www.lightstreamers.com/CELLERCISEl.htm (mini-trampoline)

www.Amazon.com/Geratherm-Basal-Mercury-Free-Thermometer/dp/B0013NB6CY (Order your own mercury-free basal thermometer, an excellent way to evaluate thyroid)

www.Amazon.com/Kitchen (Order a Vitamix blender)

Further Reading

We have touched upon a variety of helpful resources. There are a number of thyroid authors we have quoted that could be very helpful for you to review.

THESE INCLUDE OUR PREVIOUS BOOKS:
Thyroid Power
Feeling Fat, Fuzzy, or Frazzled?
The Nightingale Conspiracy
The Gift of Health
Healing with Mind Power
Energetic Approaches to Emotional Healing
Creative Imagery in Nursing

AND OTHER EXCELLENT BOOKS:
Mary Shomon, *Living Well with Graves' Disease and Hyperthyroidism*
Ridha Arem, MD, *The Thyroid Solution*
Mark Starr, MD, *Hypothyroidism Type 2*
Mark Hyman, MD, *UltraMetabolism*
William Jefferies, MD, *Safe Uses of Cortisol*
Russell T. Joffe, MD, and Anthony J. Levitt, MD, *The Thyroid Axis and Psychiatric Illness*
Gary Ross, MD, and Peter J. Bieling, PhD, *Depression and Your Thyroid*
Julia Ross, *The Mood Cure*
Elizabeth Lee Vliet, MD, *Screaming to Be Heard*
Cathryn J. Ramin, *Carved in Sand*
Steven Y. Park, MD, *Sleep, Interrupted*
Lewis E. Braverman, MD, *Diseases of the Thyroid*
Jacob Teitelbaum, MD, *From Fatigued to Fantastic!*
Dr. John Lowe, *The Metabolic Treatment of Fibromyalgia*

Georjana Shames has shared her positive, uplifting tapes and reading recommendations in her written chapter segments.

Karilee also reminds you of the enormous value of keeping spiritual books nearby, and reaching for them regularly. Such books can include popular titles, old and new. Following is a list of some of her favorite books and authors:

Kahlil Gibran, *The Prophet*

Viktor Frankl, *Man's Search for Meaning*

Scott Ohlgren, *Cellular Cleansing Made Easy*

Byron Katie, author of books and tapes about positive thinking

Carolyn Myss, author of books and tapes about energy healing

Larry Dossey, MD, author of many books about prayer and
consciousness

Barbara Dossey, RN, PhD, prolific Nightingale Scholar and
mentor to nurses

In addition, Karilee personally recommends the online radio show on Full Power Living Radio, produced by Ilene Dillon, MFT, which focuses on all things spiritual.

Full Power Living (FPL), created and hosted by Ilene Dillon, has aired on the Internet since 2004 and is awakening the world to the power and importance of human emotions. FPL explores her ideas, research, or transformational methods.

Every area of life is investigated, including business, childrearing, catastrophe, medicine, creativity, personal growth, emotions, death and dying, humor, aging, spirituality, and manifestation. Available on iTunes ("Ilene Dillon"), FPL airs live on Thursdays, 9 a.m. PT. www.emotionalpro .com. Toll-free call-in (800–630–7858) and real-time online chat for listeners.

Ilene L. Dillon, a.k.a. The Emotional Pro, is an internationally recognized radio host, author, professional speaker, coach, and longtime psychotherapist. You can reach her at ilene@emotionalpro.com.

There are so many more. Ask your friends, share books or ideas, and keep moving your goals forward.

Notes and References

(In order of citation in the book)

Chapter 1

Feit, H. "Thyroid Function in the Elderly." *Clinical Gerontological Medicine* 4 (1988):151–61.

Ditkoff, B., and P. Lo Gerfo. Columbia Presbyterian Thyroid Center. *The Thyroid Guide.* New York: HarperCollins, 2000.

Ridgeway, E. C. "Clinical Management Conference Statement." In *Hypothyroidism: The Hidden Challenge.* Denver: University of Colorado School of Medicine, 1996.

Hofman, A. "The Rotterdam Study: 2010 Objectives and Design Update." *European Journal of Epidemiology* 24, no. 9 (2009):553–72. doi:10.1007/s10654-009-9386-z. (Thyroid abnormality was determined by this study to be a separate independent risk factor for heart disease and stroke in 2001.)

Patrick, L. "Thyroid Disruption: Mechanism and Clinical Implications in Human Health." *Alternative Medicine Review* 14 (2009):326–46.

Arem, R., MD. *The Thyroid Solution.* (New York: Ballantine Books, 2000), 13–19.

Kathol, R., and J. Delahunt. "The Relationship of Anxiety and Depression to Symptoms of Hyperthyroidism." *General Hospital Psychiatry* 8 (1986):23–28.

Carson, R. *Silent Spring.* New York: Houghton Mifflin Co., 1962.

Colborn, T., et al. *Our Stolen Future.* New York: Dutton/Penguin, 1996.

Krimsky, S. *Hormonal Chaos.* Baltimore: The Johns Hopkins University Press, 2000.

Maciocia, G. *The Foundations of Chinese Medicine.* 2nd ed. London: Churchill Livingstone, 1989.

Chapter 2

Dratman, M., et al. "Iodothyronine Homeostasis in Rat Brain during Hypo- and Hyperthyroidism." *American Journal of Physiology* 245, no. 2 (1983):185–93.

Joffe, R. *The Thyroid Axis and Psychiatric Illness.* (Washington, DC: American Psychiatric Press, Inc., 1993), 45.

Hall, R., et al. "Physical Illness Manifesting as Psychiatric Disease: Analysis of a State Hospital Inpatient Population." *Archives of General Psychiatry* 37 (1980):989–95.

Davis, A. "Psychotic States Associated with Disorders of Thyroid Function." *International Journal of Psychiatry and Medicine* 19, no. 1 (1989):47–56.

Weiner, H. *Psychobiology and Human Disease.* New York: Elsevier Press, 1977.

Mason, J. "A Review of Psychoendocrine Research on the Pituitary-Thyroid System." *Psychosomatic Medicine* 30 (1968):666–81.

Baruch, P., et al. "Increased TSH Response to TRH in Refractory-Depressed Women." *American Journal of Psychiatry* 142 (1985):145–46.

Hatotani, N., et al. "Clinical and Experimental Studies on the Pathogenesis of Depression." *Psychoneuroendocrinology* 2, no. 2 (1977):115–30.

Gewirtz, G., et al. "Occult Thyroid Dysfunction in Patients with Refractory Depression." *American Journal of Psychiatry* 145, no. 8 (1988):1012–14.

Gull, W. "On a Cretinoid State Supervening in Adult Life in Women." *Transactions of the Clinical Society of London*, vol. 7. (London: Longmans, Green, and Co., 1874), 180–85.

Nemeroff, C. "Clinical Significance of Psychoneuroendocrinology in Psychiatry: Focus on the Thyroid and Adrenal." *Journal of Clinical Psychiatry* 50 (1989): 13–20.

Arem, R., MD, *The Thyroid Solution*. (New York: Ballantine Books, 2000) 6–7.

Heinrich, T., MD, and Grahm, G., MD. "Hypothyroidism Presenting as Psychosis: Myxedema Madness Revisited." *Journal of Clinical Psychiatry Primary Care Companion* 5, no. 6 (2003):260–66.

Chapter 4

World Health Organization. *Investing in Mental Health*. Produced by the Department of Mental Health and Substance Dependence, Noncommunicable Diseases and Mental Health, World Health Organization, Geneva, 2003.

Costa, E., et al. "Overview of the Field." *Metabolism* 54, no. 5 (2005):S5–S9.

Westly, E. "Different Shades of Blue: Depression Comes in Many Hues." *Scientific American Mind*, May–June 2010, 30–37.

Harrison, P. "Antidepressants Linked to Increased Risk for Death, Stroke in Postmenopausal Women." *Medscape Medical News*, December 22, 2009.

Ross, G., MD, and Peter J. Bieling, PhD. *Depression and Your Thyroid: What You Need to Know*. Oakland, CA: New Harbinger Publications, Inc., 2006.

Writing Group for the Women's Health Initiative Investigators. "Risks and Benefits of Estrogen Plus Progestin in Healthy Postmenopausal Women: Principal Results from the Women's Health Initiative Randomized Controlled Trial." *JAMA* 288, no. 3 (2002):321–333. doi:10.1001/jama.288.3.321. PMID 12117397

Joffe, R., and A. Levitt. *The Thyroid Axis and Psychiatric Illness*. Washington, DC: American Psychiatric Press, Inc., 2005.

Lowe, J. *The Metabolic Treatment of Fibromyalgia*. Boulder, CO: McDowell Publishing, 2000.

Kirsch, I. *The Emperor's New Drugs*. New York: Basic Books, 2010.

Flora, C. "The Serotonin Skeptic." *Discover Presents The Brain*, Spring 2010, 68–69.

Hendrick, V., et al. "Psychoneuroendocrinology of Mood Disorders." *Psychiatric Clinics of North America* 21, no. 2 (1998):277–92.

Savage, G. H. "Myxedema and Its Nervous Symptoms." *Journal of Mental Science* 25 (1880):417. (*Myxedema* was a word for hypothyroidism at that time.)

Murray, G. R. "Note on the Treatment of Myxedema by Hypodermic Injection of an Extract of the Thyroid Gland of a Sheep." *British Medical Journal* 2 (1891):796.

Weiner, H. "Emotions and Mentation." *The Thyroid*. 4th ed. S. C. Werner and S. H. Ingbar, eds. (New York: Harper & Row Publishers, 1987), 911.

Walker, S. *Psychiatric Signs and Symptoms Due to Medical Problems*. (Springfield, IL: Charles C. Thomas, 1967), 45.

Braverman, L., and R. Utiger. In *Werner and Ingbar's The Thyroid: A Fundamental and Clinical Text*. 5th ed. Lippincott Williams & Wilkins, 9th ed., 2004.

Smith, R. M., et al. "Effects of Thyroid State on Brain Development: Beta-Adrenergic Receptors and 5'-Nucleotidase Activity." *Brain Research* 198 (1980):375–87.

Morton, J. "Sodium Liothyronine in Metabolic Insufficiency Syndrome and Associated Disorders." *JAMA* 165 (1957):124–29.

Gewirtz, G., et al. "Occult Thyroid Dysfunction in Patients with Refractory Depression." *American Journal of Psychiatry* 145, no. 8 (1988):1012–14.

Loosen, P., and A. Prange. "Serum Thyrotropin Response to Thyrotropin-Releasing Hormone in Psychiatric Patients: A Review." *American Journal of Psychiatry* 139 (1982):405–16.

Nichols, A., and R. Ruffolo. "Functions Mediated by Alpha-Adrenoceptors." In *Alpha-Adrenoceptors: Molecular Biology, Biochemistry and Pharmacology* by K. Basel. (Basel, Switzerland: Karger, 1991), 113–79.

Gross, G. "Decreased Number of Beta-Adrenoceptors in Cerebral Cortex of Hypothroid Rats." *European Pharmacology* 61, no. 2 (1980):191–94.

Gross, G. "Reduced Number of Alpha2-Adrenoceptors in Cortical Brain Membranes of Hypothyroid Rats." *Journal of Pharmacy and Pharmacology* 33, no. 8 (1981):552.

Prange, A. "Enhancement of Imipramine Antidepressant Activity by Thyroid Hormone." *American Journal of Psychiatry* 126 (1969):39–51.

Schwark, W. "Thyroid Hormone Control of Serotonin in Developing Rat Brain." *Research Communications in Chemical Pathology and Pharmacology* 10 (1975):37.

Tejani-Butt, S. "Time Course of Altered Thyroid States on 5-HT1A Receptors and 5-HT Uptake Sites in Rat Brain." *Neuroendocrinology* 57 (1993):1011–18.

Assad, M. "Modulation in Vitro Monoamine Oxidase Activity by Thyroid Hormones." *Biochemical Pharmacology* 27 (1978):751–56.

Goodwin, F. "Potentiation of Antidepressive Effects of Thyronine (T3) in Tricyclic Antidepressant Nonresponders." *American Journal of Psychiatry* 139 (1982):34.

Surks, M. "A New Radioimmunoassay for Plasma L-thyronine: Measurements in Thyroid Disease and in Patients Maintained on Hormonal Replacement." *Journal of Clinical Investigation* 51 (1972):3104–13.

Prange, A. "Enhancement of the Imipramine Antidepressant Activity by Thyroid Hormone." *American Journal of Psychiatry* 126 (1969):457–59.

Wilson, I., et al. "Thyroid Hormone Enhancement of Imipramine in Nonretarded Depression." *New England Journal of Medicine* 282 (1970):1063–67.

Coppen, A., et al. "Comparative Antidepressant Value of L-Tryptophan and Imipramine With and Without Attempted Potentiation by Liothyronine." *Archives of General Psychiatry* 26 (1972):234–41.

Wheathley, D. "Potentiation of Amytripthaline by Thyroid Hormone." *Archives of General Psychiatry* 26 (1972):229–33.

Thase, N., et al. "Treatment of Imipramine-Resistant Recurrent Depression: An Open Clinical Trial of Adjunctive Tri-iodothyronine." *Journal of Clinical Psychiatry* 50 (1989):385–88.

Whybrow, P. C. In *Werner and Ingbar's The Thyroid: A Fundamental and Clinical Text.* 5th ed. Lippincott Williams & Wilkins, 9th ed., 2004.

Goodwin, F., et al. "Potentiation of Antidepressant Effects by Tri-iodothyronine in Tricyclic Nonresponders." *American Journal of Psychiatry* 139 (1982):34–38.

Schwarcz, G., et al. "Normal Thyroid Function in Desimapramine Nonresponders Compared to Responders by the Addition of Tri-iodothyronine." *American Journal of Psychiatry* 141 (1984):1614–16.

Maciocia, G. *The Foundations of Chinese Medicine.* 2nd ed. (London: Churchill Livingstone, 1989), 73.

Chödrön, P. *When Things Fall Apart: Heart Advice for Difficult Times.* Also, *Choosing a Fresh Alternative.* (You can purchase her books and tapes at www.shambhala.org/teachers/pema/bookstore2.php.)

Chapter 5

Kessler, R., et al. "Lifetime and Twelve-Month Prevalence of DSM-III-R Psychiatric Disorders in the US: Results from the National Co-morbidity Study." *Archives of General Psychiatry* 51 (1994):8–19.

Lindermann, C., et al. "Thyroid Dysfunction in Phobic Patients." *Psychosomatics* 25 (1984):603–606.

Frisch, N., and L. Frisch. *Psychiatric Mental Health Nursing.* 2nd ed. Albany, NY: Delmar Press/Thomson Learning, 2002.

Graves, R. "Clinical Lectures." *London Medicine and Surgery Journal* 7 (1835):516.

Wartofsky, L., et al. "Diseases of the Thyroid." *Harrison's Principles of Internal Medicine.* 12th ed. (New York: McGraw-Hill, 1991), 1692–1712.

Katerndahl, D., and L. Van de Creek. "Hyperthyroidism and Panic Attacks." *Journal of Psychosomatics* 24 (1983):491–96.

Raj, A., and D. Sheehan. "Medical Evaluation of Panic Attacks." *Journal of Clinical Psychiatry* 48 (1987):309–13.

Cathol, R. "Depression and Anxiety Associated with Hyperthyroidism." *Psychosomatics* 27 (1986):501–505.

Stein, M. "Panic Disorder and Medical Illness." *Psychosomatics* 27 (1986):833–40.

Thompson, W., et al. "Low Basal Metabolism Following Thyrotoxicosis." *Journal of Clinical Investigation* 5 (1928):471–501.

Landsberg, L., and J. Axelrod. "Influence of Pituitary, Thyroid, and Adrenal Hormones on Norepinephrine Metabolism." *Circulation Research* 22, no. 5 (1968):559–71.

Iranmanish, A., et al. "Dynamics of 24-Hour Endogenous Cortisol Secretion and Clearance in Primary Hypothyroidism Assessed Before and After Partial Thyroid Hormone Replacement." *Journal of Clinical Endocrinology and Metabolism* 70 (1990):155.

de Groot, L., et al. *The Thyroid and Its Diseases.* 5th ed. (New York: John Wiley & Sons, 1984), 574–77.

Ungar, A., et al. "Regulation of the Adrenal Medulla." *Physiology Review* 63 (1983):787–843.

Goldberg, M. "Diagnosis of Euthyroid Hypometabolism." *American Journal of Obstetrics and Gynecology* 81, no. 5 (1961):1057–58.

Kamilaris, T., et al. "Effect of Altered Thyroid Levels on Hypothalamic-Pituitary Adrenal Function." *Journal of Clinical Endocrinology and Metabolism* 65 (1987):994–99.

Atterwill, C., et al. "Effects of Thyroid Status on Presynaptic Alpha2-Adrenoceptor Function and Beta-adrenoceptor Binding in the Rat Brain." *Journal of Neural Transmission* 59 (1984):43–55.

Felten, D., et al. "Noradrenergic Sympathetic Neural Interactions with the Immune System." *Immunological Reviews* 100 (1987):225–60.

DeBoel, S., et al. "Thyroid Hormone Reserve in Asymptomatic Autoimmune Thyroiditis." *Acta Endocrinologica* (Copenhagen) 114 (1987):336–39.

Fundaro, A., and L. Molinengo. "Emotional Behavior in Relation to Hypothyroidism and Hyperthyroidism." *Medical Sciences Research* 15 (1987):253–54.

Kosten, T., et al. "The Dexamethazone Suppression Test and Thyrotropin-Releasing Hormone Stimulation Test in Post-Traumatic Stress Disorder." *Biological Psychiatry* 28 (1990):657–64.

Kauffman, C., et al. "Biological Markers of Affective Disorders and Post-Traumatic Stress Disorder." *Journal of Clinical Psychiatry* 48 (1994):132–37.

Stein, M., and T. Uhde. "Thyrotropin and Prolactin Responses to Protirelin (TRH) Prior to and During Chronic Imipramine Treatment in Patients with Panic Disorder." *Psycho-neuroendocrinology* 15 (1990):381–89.

George, D., et al. "Effect of Pregnancy on Panic Attacks." *American Journal of Psychiatry* 144 (1987):1078–79.

Metz, A., et al. "Postpartum Panic Disorder." *Journal of Clinical Psychiatry* 49 (1988):278–79.

Shomon, M. *Living Well with Graves' Disease and Hyperthyroidism.* New York: Harper Paperbacks, 2005.

Moore, E. *Graves' Disease: A Practical Guide.* Jefferson, NC: McFarland & Company, 2001.

Chapter 6

Riven, A. "Alzheimer's as Seen by a Doctor Who Suddenly Finds Himself a Patient." Outside contributor article for the *Los Angeles Times*, July 1, 2010.

Arem, R., MD. *The Thyroid Solution.* (New York: Ballantine Books, 2000), 58.

Montauk, S., et al. "Attention Deficit Hyperactivity Disorder." *eMedicine Specialties/Medscape.* http://emedicine.medscape.com/. Updated February 22, 2010.

Hayslip, C., et al. "The Value of Serum Antimicrosomal Antibody Testing in Screening for Symptomatic Postpartum Thyroid Dysfunction." *American Journal of Obstetrics and Gynecology* 159 (1988):203–209.

Fierro-Benitez, R. "Long-Term Effects of Correction of Iodine Deficiency on Intellectual Development." *Proceedings of the 5th Meeting of the PAHO/WHO Technical Group on Endemic Goiter and Iodine Deficiency.* Washington, DC: Pan-American Health Organization, 1986.

Haggerty, J., et al. "Subclinical Hypothyroidism: A Review of Neuropsychiatric Aspects." *International Journal of Psychiatry in Medicine* 20, no. 2 (1990):193–208.

Dawes, B. "Neurological and Cognitive Function." In *Gerontologic Nursing.* (St. Louis: C.V. Mosby Publishers), 727–66.

Oppenheim, G. "The Earliest Signs of Alzheimer's Disease." *Journal of Geriatric Psychiatry and Neurology* 7 (1994):116–20.

Frisch, N., and L. Frisch. *Psychiatric Mental Health Nursing.* 2nd ed. (Albany, NY: Delmar Press/Thomson Learning, 2002), 568.

Joffe, R., and A. Levitt. *The Thyroid Axis and Psychiatric Illness.* (Washington, DC: American Psychiatric Press, Inc., 2005), 46.

Haggerty, J., et al. "Organic Brain Syndrome Associated with Marginal Hypothyroidism." *American Journal of Psychiatry* 143 (1986):785–86.

Fader, B., and F. Struve. "The Possible Value of the Electroencephalogram (EEG) in Detecting Subclinical Hypothyroidism." *Clinical Electroencephalography* 3 (1972):94–101.

Lowe, J. *The Metabolic Treatment of Fibromyalgia.* (Boulder, CO: McDowell Publishing, 2000), 588.

Oppenheimer, J. "Thyroid Hormone Action at the Molecular Level." In *Werner and Ingbar's The Thyroid: A Fundamental and Clinical Text.* 6th ed., 204–24.

Schmidt, R. "Integrative Functions of the Central Nervous System." *Fundamentals of Neurophysiology.* 3rd ed. (New York: Springer-Verlag, 1985), 270–316.

Berne, R., and M. Levy. *Principles of Physiology.* (St. Louis: C.V. Mosby Co., 1990), 170.

Stevens, J., and M. Killeen. "A Randomised Controlled Trial Testing the Impact of Exercise on Cognitive Symptoms and Disability of Residents with Dementia." *Journal of Mental Health Nursing* 21, no. 1 (2006):32–40.

Chapter 7

Kamel, N. S., and J. K. Gammack. "Insomnia in the Elderly: Cause, Approach, and Treatment." *American Journal of Medicine* 119, no. 6 (2006): 463–69.

Nutter, Dennis, Jr., MD, et al. "Sleep Disorder, Problems Associated with Other Disorders." *eMedicine News Online.* http://emedicine.medscape.com. February 18, 2010.

Hertz, G., PhD, ABSM. "Sleep Dysfunction in Women." *eMedicine News Online.* http:// emedicine.medscape.com. Updated December 15, 2008.

Barclay, L., MD, "Medication for Insomnia or Anxiety Linked to 36% Increase in Mortality Risk." Medscape CME Clinical Briefs, October 5, 2010. www.medscapecme.com

Shomon, M. *Living Well with Graves' Disease and Hyperthyroidism.* (New York: HarperCollins, 2005), 54.

Ross, J. *The Mood Cure.* (New York: Viking, 2002), 232.

Starr, M., MD. *Hypothyroidism Type 2: The Epidemic.* (Columbia, MO: The Mark Starr Trust, 2007), 249.

Arem, R., MD, *The Thyroid Solution.* (New York: Ballantine Books, 2000) 39.

Rothfield, G., and D. Romaine. *Thyroid Balance.* (Avon, MA: Adams Media Corporation, 2003), 14.

Park, S., MD. *Sleep, Interrupted.* New York: Jodev Press, LLC, 2008.

Weinstock, W., et al. "Blockade of 5-Hydroxytriptamine Receptors in Central Nervous System by Beta-Adrenoceptor Antagonists." *Neuropharmacology* 16 (1977):273.

Morgane, P. "Serotonin: 20 Years Later—Monoamine Theory of Sleep: The Role of Serotonin: A Review." *Psychopharmacology Bulletin* 17 (1981):13–17.

Soszynski, P., et al. "The Circadian Rhythm of Melatonin in Hypothyroidism and Hyperthyroidism." *Acta Endocrinologica* 119, no. 2 (1988):240–44.

Bals-Pratsch, M., et al. "Episodic Variations of Prolactin, Thyroid-Stimulating Hormone, Luteinizing Hormone, Melatonin and Cortisol in Infertile Women with Subclinical Hypothyroidism." *Human Reproduction* 12, no. 5 (1997):896–904.

Schafer, R. "Clinical Biomechanics." Chapter in *Musculoskeletal Actions and Reactions.* 2nd ed. Baltimore: Williams and Wilkins, 1987.

Luden, A., et al. "The Recuperative Effects of REM Sleep and Stage 4 Sleep on Human Performance after Complete Sleep Loss." *Psychophysiology* 11 (1974):133–36.

Kok, S., et al. "Serial Measurements of TSH Determinations in Normal and Narcoleptic Sleep." *American Journal of Physiology—Endocrinology and Metabolism* 288 (December 2005):892–99.

Deadman, H. *A Manual of Acupuncture,* (often quoted rare book; publisher/place of publication not available) 2001, 337.

Chapter 8

WrongDiagnosis.com. http://www.wrongdiagnosis.com/ (Accessed June 16, 2010).

National Institute on Drug Abuse (NIDA), division of the National Institutes of Health (NIH). http://www.drugabuse.gov, accessed June 18, 2010.

Frisch, N., and L. Frisch. *Psychiatric Mental Health Nursing.* 2nd ed. (Albany, NY: Delmar Press/Thomson Learning, 2002), 436.

Ross, J. *The Diet Cure.* New York: Penguin Books, 1999. Also, *The Mood Cure.*

Arem, R., MD. *The Thyroid Solution.* New York: Ballantine Books, 2000.

Gambert, S., et al. "Thyroid Hormone Regulation of Central Nervous System (CNS) Beta-endorphin and ACTH." *Hormone Metabolic Research* 12 (1980): 345–46.

Donhoffer, S., and J. Vonotzky. "The Effect of Thyroxine on Food Intake and Selection." *American Journal of Physiology* 150 (1947):334–39.

Hyman, M. *UltraMetabolism*. (New York: Scribner, 2006), 177.

Vliet, E. L., MD. *Screaming to Be Heard: Hormonal Connections Women Suspect and Doctors Ignore.* New York: M. Evans & Co., Inc., 1995.

Ilias, I., et al. "Thyroid Function of Former Opioid Addicts on Naltrexone Treatment." *Acta Medica* 44, no. 1 (2001):33–35.

Milam, J. *Under the Influence.* Seattle: Madrone Press, 1981.

Fukayama, H., et al. "Examination of Antithyroid Effects of Smoking Products in Cultured Thyroid Follicles." *Acta Endocrinologica* (Copenhagen) 127, no. 6 (December 1992):520–25.

Hyman, *UltraMetabolism*, 185.

Jefferies, W. *Safe Uses of Cortisol.* Revised ed. Springfield, IL: Charles C. Thomas, 2004.

Joffe, R., and A. Levitt. *The Thyroid Axis and Psychiatric Illness.* Washington, DC: American Psychiatric Press, Inc., 2005.

Chapter 9

Zois, C., et al. "High Prevalence of Autoimmune Thyroiditis in Schoolchildren after Elimination of Iodine Deficiency in Northwestern Greece." *Thyroid* 13 (December 2003):1187.

Lentsch, E., et al. "Induction of Papillary Thyroid Cancer in Animals by the Administration of High-Dose Iodine." *eMedicine Specialties*, Head and Neck Surgery. http://emedicine.medscape.com/specialities. April 24, 2009.

The Yellow Emperor's Inner Classic. San Francisco: Shambala Press, 1995. (This ancient text is believed by many scholars to have been written and printed in the first century B.C.E. Although it is attributed to Huang Di, the Yellow Emperor, historians believe multiple authors' work was compiled during the Han Dynasty [206 B.C.E.–220 C.E.] into one book known as the Yellow Emperor's Inner Classic.)

Chapter 10

Golomb, B. "Chocolate Consumption in Individuals with Depressive Symptoms: A Cross-sectional Study." *Archives of Internal Medicine* 170 (March 2010):699–703.

Keegan, G. T., MD, and L. Keegan, RN, PhD. *Healing Waters.* New York: Berkley Publishing/Penguin, 1998.

Shames, Richard, and Chuck Sterin. *Healing with Mind Power.* Emmaus, PA: Rodale Press, 1978.

Index

Underscored references indicate boxed text or tables.

A

Acetylcholine, 146
Acetyl-cholinesterase inhibitors, 147
ActivEssentials, 92
Acupuncture, 221–23. *See also*
    Complementary healing
ADD and ADHD, 139–40, 141–42
Addiction and substance abuse, 193–97,
    205–6, 257–58
Adrenal function, 127, 128, 162–63,
    220–21
Aging, 7, 139, 142, 145, 160
Air filters, 242
Alzheimer's disease, 139, 146
Amino acids, 67, 200, 206, 261, 263
Anger. *See* Irritability and anger
Anorexia. *See* Eating disorders
Antidepressants
    for anxiety relief, 121
    boosted by thyroid hormone, 87, 90
    cautions and dangers, 78, 93
    ineffectiveness of, 29, 78, 80
    MAO inhibitors, 88
    misdiagnosis for, 10
    number of people taking, 77
    sleep disorders and, 171
    SSRIs, 78, 121
    thyroid hormone as, 80
Antioxidants, 66–67, 261, 262
Anxiety and fear
    action plan for, 134–35
    affects on self and others, 115–17
    biochemistry of, 120–22
    bottom line for, 133–34
    common with thyroid disease, 44
    control patterns with, 114–15
    definitions of terms, 112
    with low thyroid, 40–41, 118–19,
        119–20
    panic disorder, 112, 113, 123
    pharmacologic drugs for, 121
    post-traumatic stress disorder, 123
    prevalence of, 111, 115
    stages of anxiety, 112–13
    stories, 31–32, 37–38
    telltale behaviors, 113–14
    treatment for, 124–31
    variations of symptoms, 113–14
Aricept (donepezil), 147
Armour thyroid, 96–97, 103, 262
Ashwaganda, 200, 206, 263
Attention deficit disorders (ADD or
    ADHD), 139–40, 141–42
Authenticity, 269
Autoimmune support, 213
Autoimmune thyroid imbalance, 40, 122,
    148, 174, 218
Awareness, 270

B

Basal metabolic rate, 59, 60
Benzodiazepines, 121
Beta-adrenaline receptors, 86–87
Beta-blockers, 121
BioPure Protein, 67, 261
Bipolar disorder, 43, 77
Bladder Meridian, 23–24
Bodywork, 252–54
Brain
    activity during sleep, 166–67
    energy used by, 33
    meridian theory and, 47, 48, 49
    sluggish, treating, 90–91
    thyroid and function of, 10–11, 33–34,
        39–40, 43–44, 79–80, 146–47
    thyroid hormone activity not
        measurable in, 40
Bulimia. *See* Eating disorders
BuSpar, 121

C

Calcium, 211–12, 224
Canary Club website, 44, 54, 220, 273
Carnosic acid, 90–91
Ceralin, 152
Chewable Digestion, 214

Chromium, 212, 224
Cleansing activities, 237, 266
Coenzyme Q_{10} (CoQ_{10}), 92
Coffea Cruda, 175, 183, 263
Cognition, 142
Cognitive dysfunction, 143
Complementary healing
  acupuncture, 221–23
  for diagnosis, 67–70
  for Edgy mind-type, 131–33
  Five Elements theory, 100
  for Foggy mind-type, 154–56
  lifestyle choices, 256–58
  meridian theory, 22–24, 47–49
  mind/body integration in, 21–22,
    24–25
  for Moody mind-type, 100–102
  for Needy mind-type, 202–5
  for Sleepy mind-type, 179–82
Compounded thyroxine, 200–201, 206
Compulsion, 112
Conception Meridian, 24
Congee (rice pudding), 101
Control patterns with anxiety, 114–15
CoQ-10 ST 100, 92
Creativity, 269
Cytomel (liothyronine), 153, 157, 177,
  262

D

D_3 1000, 91, 103
Dear Thyroid website, 32
Deep tissue work, 253
Dementia, 139, 145–51
Depression
  action plan for, 103
  biochemical view of, 85
  bottom line for, 102–3
  low thyroid linked to, 42–43, 44,
    77–78, 79, 83–85
  postpartum, 48, 81–82
  prevalence of, 77
  serotonin/thyroid interaction and, 87
  severity of low thyroid and, 84–85
  supplements helping with, 216–17
  treatment for, 48, 87, 88, 89–102
Desiccated thyroid, 94–99, 262
Diagnosis. *See also* Tests
  action plan for, 71
  Acupuncture theory for, 67–70
  family history for, 57–58

physical signs for, 57, 59
physical symptoms for, 57
psychological symptoms for, 57
questionnaires for, 60, 62–66
temperature taking for, 59–60
Digest Chewables, 214
Digestive enzymes, 212–13, 224
Discernment, 268
DNA, thyroid connection to, 33
Doctors, working with, 274–78
Donepezil (Aricept), 147

E

Eating disorders, 186–93, 198–99, 205
EcoNugenics, 280
Edgy mind-type. *See also* Anxiety and
      fear; Irritability and anger
  action plan for, 134–35
  affects on self and others, 115–17
  avoiding energy drainers, 110
  bottom line for, 133–34
  categories of edginess, 111–12
  definitions of terms, 112
  family behavior patterns and, 106–9
  minimizing stress, 108–10
  obsessive-compulsive disorder, 112
  science of, 118–19
  stakes for, 111
  stories, 105–6, 108
  supplements for, 216
  treatment for, 124–33
Energenics, 206, 263
Energy drainers, 110, 266–67
Enzymes, Inc., 280
Enzyme support, 212–13, 224
Estrogen, 219
Exercise
  action plan for, 261
  complementary healing, 257
  for Edgy mind-type, 133
  for Foggy mind-type, 156
  for Moody mind-type, 102
  for Needy mind-type, 204
  overview, 248–52
  for Sleepy mind-type, 181

F

Family history, 15, 57–58, 65, 106–9,
    121
Fear, 112. *See also* Anxiety and fear
FFI (fatal familial insomnia), 166

Fibrozym, 215
5-HTP, 92–93, 176, 183
Five Elements theory, 100
Fluoridated water, 240–42
Foggy mind-type
    action plan for, 157
    ADD or ADHD, 139–42
    bottom line for, 157
    dementia, 139, 145–51
    memory difficulties, 139, 142–45,
        151–52, 156
    Nora's story, 137–38
    postpartum mind issues, 144–45
    stakes for, 139
    supplements for, 215
    T3 thyroid hormone for, 152–53
    treatment for, 151–52, 154–56
Formula 50, 216
Formulas from Enzymes, Inc., 212–13,
    214
Free T3 tests, 54, 153, 274
Free T4 tests, 46, 54, 86, 153, 274

G

Gallbladder Meridian, 24
Gastro Calm, 214
Generalized anxiety disorder, 112
Gifts, using yours, 267–71
Gingko biloba, 152
GingkoRose, 152
Glutamine, 200
Governing Meridian, 24
Gratitude, 270–71
Graves' antibody tests, 129, 135
Graves' disease, 128, 129, 135
Guggulsterone, 151–52, 157, 262

H

Hashimoto's thyroiditis, 129, 139
Health care options, 226–27
Heart Meridian, 23, 69, 100–102
Hep-Forte, 216
HER AdvancedPlus Panel, 54, 274
Herbal sleep medications, 175–76
High thyroid. See hyperthyroidism
Histame, 216–17
Homeopathic remedies, 175
Honesty, 269–70
Hops, 175, 183

Hungry humans, 266–67
Hyperthyroidism (high thyroid). See also
        Thyroid imbalance
    early research in, 40
    edginess due to, 118–19
    as Kidney Yin deficiency, 47, 69
    questionnaire for, 63–64
    science of, 118–19
    sleep disorders with, 162, 164–65,
        169–70
    symptoms of, 9, 11, 40–41, 63–64
    treatment for, 41, 125–26, 128–31
Hypothyroidism (low thyroid). See also
        Thyroid imbalance
    aging and increase in, 145
    anxiety due to, 40–41, 118–19, 119–20
    brain function and, 146–47
    depression linked to, 42–43, 44, 77–78,
        79, 83–85
    female problems due to, 9
    as Kidney Yang deficiency, 47, 69
    low mood linked to, 85–86
    Lucy Johnson's story, 51–52
    mechanisms impacting mood,
        86–88
    memory difficulties with, 143, 144
    obesity associated with, 191
    physical symptoms of, 86
    postpartum, 144–45
    questionnaire for, 62–63
    severe, 84–85
    sleep disorders with, 162, 165,
        169–73
    subclinical, 42–43
    symptoms of, 9, 42–43, 62–63
    treatment for, 90–99, 124–28

I

Immune system
    autoimmune thyroid imbalance, 40,
        122, 148, 150, 174, 218
    noradrenaline as regulator of, 122
    surge after childbirth, 81–82
Insomnia. See Sleep disorders
Integrity, 269–70
Iodine, 143, 144, 217–18
Iron, 211–12, 224
Irritability and anger
    anxiety exhibited as, by men, 113
    stories, 15–16, 18–19, 31–32

supplements helping with, 216–17
thyroid imbalance causing, 122–23
Iso D$_3$, 91, 262

K

Kidney Meridian, 24, 47, 48, 69, 179–81

L

Lacidofil DF, 215
Lady's slipper, 175, 183
Large Intestine Meridian, 22
L-carnitine, 125
Levothroid, 97, 126–28
Levothyroxine, 126–28, 134, 177, 206,
    262, 263
Levoxyl, 126–28
Licorice, 213, 224
Lifestyle choices. *See also* Exercise
    action plan for, 259–60
    air filtering, 242
    bodywork, 252–54
    bottom line for, 258–59
    cleansing activities, 237
    complementary healing, 256–58
    for Edgy mind-type, 133
    for Foggy mind-type, 156
    fundamentals of, 228–31
    for Moody mind-type, 101–2
    for Needy mind-type, 204–5
    nutrition, 231–36
    parasite eradication, 238–40
    self-care suggestions, 237–38
    spiritual awareness, 254–55
    stress reduction, 243–48
    water considerations, 240–42
Liothyronine (Cytomel), 153, 157, 177,
    262
Lipoic acid, 126
Lipotain, 152, 157, 262
Liver Meridian, 24, 69, 131–32
Low thyroid. *See* Hypothyroidism
L-tryptophan, 176, 183
Lung Meridian, 22, 69, 202–4

M

Magnesium, 212, 224
Maintenance program. *See also* Lifestyle
    choices
    action plan, 224
    bottom line, 223

complementary healing, 221–23
health care options, 226–27
nutritional support, 210–18
rebalancing other hormones, 219–21
Mania with high thyroid, 41
MAO inhibitors, 88
Massage, 252–54
MedCaps T3, 125, 134, 175, 183, 262
Medizym, 216
Melatonin, 170, 176–77, 183
Memantine (Namenda), 147
MemorAll, 152
Memory difficulties, 139, 142–45, 151–52,
    156
Mentalin, 206, 263
Metabolism, 66–67, 87, 193–96
Metagenics, Inc., 279
Methimazole (Tapazole), 129, 130, 135
Minerals, 66, 211–12
Mint tea, 132
Moody mind-type. *See also* Depression
    action plan for, 103
    bottom line for, 102–3
    mechanisms impacting mood, 86–88
    Rosie's story, 75–76
    stakes for, 76–77
    treatment for, 90–102
Multigenics vitamins, 66, 261
Multivitamins, 66, 92, 261
Musculoskeletal support, 215–16
MyoCalm P.M., 176, 183

N

Namenda (memantine), 147
Narcolepsy, 161, 174–75
Naturally Vitamins, 280
Nature-Throid, 96, 103, 262
Needy mind-type
    action plan for, 206
    bottom line for, 205–6
    eating disorders, 186–93, 198–99,
        205
    Maria's story, 185–86, 197–98
    stakes for, 186–87
    substance abuse and addiction, 187,
        193–97, 205–6, 257–58
    treatment for, 200–205
Noradrenaline, 86, 119, 122
Nurses' role, 12, 265
Nutrition, 231–36, 256–57, 260

O

Obsessive-compulsive disorder, 112
Omega EFA, 67, 261
Omega oil supplements, 67, 261
Orange peel, 175, 183
Oraxinol, 152, 157, 262
Over-the-counter remedies. *See also*
    Supplements
  for high thyroid, 125–26
  for low thyroid, 124–25
  for memory difficulties, 151–52
  for Needy mind-type, 200
  for sleep disorders, 175–77
Oxygenics, 67, 152, 261

P

Padma Basic, 214, 224
Panic disorder, 112, 113, 123. *See also*
    Anxiety and fear
Parasite eradication, 238–40
Passionflower, 175, 183
Pericardium Meridian, 24
Pharmacologic drugs, 5–6, 13–14, 21,
    29, 39, 121. *See also*
    Antidepressants
Phobia, 112. *See also* Anxiety and fear
Physical signs, 57, 59, 65–66
Physical symptoms, 5, 57, 62–64, 86
Pollution, 11–12, 29
Postpartum depression, 48, 81–82
Postpartum mind issues, 144–45
Post-traumatic stress disorder, 123
Pregnancy, 48, 81–82, 123, 144–45
Probiotics, 215, 224
Progesterone, 219–20
Proloid desiccated thyroid, 97
Psychological symptoms. *See also specific*
    mind-types
  in diagnosis process, 57
  disability due to, 77
  genetic factors in, 37
  hormonal sources of, 14–15
  limitations of drugs for, 5–6, 13
  in men, 18–19
  mind-body split and, 5
  prevalence of, 76, 77
  from thyroid problems, 10–11, 28–29,
    30, 34–36, 38–39, 40–43
  thyroid treatment healing, 17
PTU (propylthiouracil), 129, 130, 135

Q

Qec100, 92
Qi, rebalancing, 222–23
Quercetin, 125
Questionnaires, 60–66, 277–78

R

Rebalancing other hormones, 219–21
Related conditions, 57, 59, 64
Resistance to thyroid hormone, 57, 153
Retardation, thyroid linked to, 33–34
Rice pudding (congee), 101
Ritalin, 140
Rosemary extract, 90–91, 262
Rutozym, 215

S

SAM-e, 93–94
Sedalin, 176, 183
Selective serotonin reuptake inhibitors
    (SSRIs), 78, 121
Selenium, 212
Serotonin, 87, 92–93, 120, 121, 170–71, 192
Sex hormone, rebalancing, 219–20
Skullcap, 176, 183
Sleep, 165–68
Sleep disorders
  adrenaline causing, 162–63
  ease of disturbance and, 172
  FFI (fatal familial insomnia), 166
  as frequent in thyroid patients, 161–62,
    163
  muscle weakness causing, 171–72
  narcolepsy, 161, 174–75
  prevalence of, 160, 161
  protocol for, 177–79
  serotonin's role in, 170–71
  sleep apnea, 161, 169
  thyroid imbalance causing, 162,
    164–65, 168, 169–71
  thyroid imbalance due to, 169
  treatment for, 162–63, 175–77, 179–82
Sleepy mind-type
  action plan for, 183
  bottom line for, 178–79, 182
  protocol for, 177–79
  stakes for, 160–61
  stories, 159–60, 164, 172–73
  supplements for, 215
  treatment for, 162–63, 175–77, 179–82

Small Intestine Meridian, 23
Smoking, quitting, 257–58
Somnolin, 176, 183
Soy isoflavones, 126
Spiritual awareness, 254–55
Spleen Meridian, 23, 69, 101, 155
Stimulin, 216
St. John's wort, 93
Stomach Meridian, 23, 155
Stress. *See also* Edgy mind-type
    endocrine abnormalities due to, 40
    family behavior patterns and, 106–9
    reducing, 108–9, 243–48, 260–61
Subclinical hypothyroidism, 42–43
Substance abuse and addiction, 187,
    193–97, 205–6, 257–58
Supplements. *See also* Over-the-counter
        remedies
    action plan for, 224
    for autoimmune support, 213
    depression or irritability aids, 216–17
    for Edgy mind-type, 124–26, 130–31
    for enzyme support, 212–13
    for fixing sluggish metabolism,
        66–67
    for help with thyroid problems, 38
    for high thyroid, 130–31
    for low thyroid, 90–94
    for Moody mind-type, 90–94
    for musculoskeletal support, 215–16
    in regular medical care, 38
    thyroid boosting, 213
Synthroid, 96, 126–28, 177

T

T1 thyroid hormone, 95, 99
T2 thyroid hormone, 95, 99
T3 thyroid hormone, 39, 84. *See also*
        Tests; Thyroid medicines
T4 thyroid hormone, 84, 95, 99. *See also*
        Tests; Thyroid medicines
T-150 thyroid glandular, 124, 134, 262
Tapazole (methimazole), 129, 130, 135
Taurine, 200
Temperature, taking, 59–60
10 Mushroom Formula, 214
Tests. *See also specific tests*
    additional diagnostic methods, 57
    blood source for, 54, 56, 70
    dosage adjustments and, 154
    eating disorders and, 192

full thyroid evaluation, 21
    improvements needed in, 56–57
    interpreting, 55–56
    recommended panel of, 54, 274
    for resistance to thyroid hormone,
        153
    self-ordering, 44, 54–55, 273
    standard, inadequacy of, 20, 30, 42,
        46, 52, 53, 67–68, 86, 97
    telling your doctor about, 44–45, 56
    thyroid problems with normal test
        results, 30, 42, 57, 70
TG (thyroglobulin) antibody test, 54
Thermometer, using, 59–60
Thyrocalcitonin, 95
Thyroid-friendly practitioners, 274–75
Thyroid gland functions, 4, 16–17, 33, 59
Thyroid glandular, 124–25, 134, 262
Thyroid hormone. *See also* Tests; Thyroid
        medicines
    as antidepressant, 87, 88, 89–90
    biochemicals impacted by, 191
    brain function and, 10–11, 33–34,
        39–40, 43–44, 79–80
    MAO activity decreased by, 88
    resistance to, 57, 153
    serotonin interaction with, 87, 170–71
    supplements aiding, 90–94
Thyroid imbalance. *See also*
        Hyperthyroidism (high thyroid);
        Hypothyroidism (low thyroid)
    action plan for, 26
    addiction and, 195–97
    aging and increase in, 7
    autoimmune, 40, 122, 148, 150, 174,
        218
    death resulting from, 3
    eating disorders and, 188–90, 190–91,
        191–93
    epidemic of, 8, 11, 30
    genetic factors in, 194
    heart disease and stroke risk with, 8
    importance of diagnosing, 46
    inadequate treatment of, 35
    mental symptoms due to, 10–11, 28–29,
        30, 34, 38–39
    as microcosm for ills of medical
        system, 14
    mild, clinical significance of, 9, 10
    misdiagnosed or undiagnosed, 1, 3–4,
        8, 9, 10–11, 21, 35, 38–39

Thyroid imbalance *(cont.)*
   as model of biology of mood, 122
   with normal tests, 30, 42, 57, 70
   overview, 25–26
   panic disorder linked to, 123
   pollution causing, 11–12, 29
   prevalence of, 4, 7, 8
   sleep disorders causing, 169
   sleep disorders with, 162, 164–65, 168, 169–73
   stakes for, 29–30
   tremendous variability in symptoms of, 10
Thyroidinum, 175, 183, 263
Thyroid medicines. *See also* Over-the-counter remedies; Supplements
   adrenal insufficiency unmasked by, 127, 128
   antidepressants boosted by, 87, 90
   desiccated thyroid, 94–99, 262
   for Edgy mind-type, 123, 124–31
   for Foggy mind-type, 152–53
   frequency of prescription, 1, 4, 7
   going off, 97, 98–99
   long-term management of, 97–99
   monitoring, 96–97
   for Moody mind-type, 94–99
   for Needy mind-type, 200–202
   overmedication symptoms, 97
   for Sleepy mind-type, 164, 177–78
   synthetic vs. natural, 95, 96, 99
   trial for diagnosis, 19–20
Thyroid Mind Power website, 67
Thyroid Support formula, 213, 214
Thyrosol, 103, 125, 175, 183, 262
Thyroxine, 126–28, 200–201, 206
Thytrophin, 124
Tobacco addiction, 194–95

TPO (thyroid peroxidase antibody) test, 54, 274
TRH (thyroid-releasing hormone) test, 85, 86, 123
Trial of thyroid medicine, 19–20
Tryptophan, 93, 170, 176, 183
TSH (thyroid-stimulating hormone) test
   capillary vs. venous blood for, 56, 70
   change in normal range for, 8, 55
   inaccuracy of, 46, 52, 53, 86, 97
   in recommended test panel, 54, 274
   subclinical condition shown by, 42
Tyrosine, 200

U
Ultra Dophilus DF, 215
Unithroid, 126

V
Valerian root, 175, 183
Valium, 121
Vitamin D, 91, 103, 256, 262
Vitamins, 66, 92, 221, 261, 279–80

W
Water considerations, 240–42
Wellness Essentials vitamins, 92
Wes-Throid, 96
Wholeness perspective, 6–7
Women. *See also* Pregnancy
   bipolar disorder and, 77
   minimizing stress, 109–10
   postmenopausal, antidepressants and, 78
   thyroid-related female problems, 9

X
Xymogen, 279–80